Practical Digital Mammography

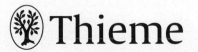

Practical Digital Mammography

Beverly E. Hashimoto, M.D., F.A.C.R.
Section Head of Ultrasound
Virginia Mason Medical Center
Assistant Clinical Professor of Radiology
University of Washington
Seattle, Washington

Thieme
New York • Stuttgart

Thieme Medical Publishers, Inc.
333 Seventh Ave.
New York, NY 10001

Associate Editor: Birgitta Brandenburg
Assistant Editor: Ivy Ip
Vice President, Production and Electronic Publishing: Anne T. Vinnicombe
Production Editor: Print Matters, Inc.
Managing Editor: Owen Zurhellen IV
Vice President, International Marketing: Cornelia Schulze
Associate Marketing Director: Verena Diem
Chief Financial Officer: Peter van Woerden
President: Brian D. Scanlan
Compositor: Compset, Inc.
Printer: The Maple-Vail Book Manufacturing Group

Library of Congress Cataloging-in-Publication Data

Hashimoto, Beverly.
   Practical digital mammography / Beverly E. Hashimoto.
     p. ; cm.
   Includes bibliographical references and index.
   ISBN 978-1-58890-620-5 (Americas : alk. paper)—ISBN 978-3-13-148041-5 (rest of world : alk. paper)
     1. Breast—Radiography—Case studies.   2. Breast—Diseases—Diagnosis—Case studies.   I. Title.
     [DNLM: 1. Mammography—methods—Case Reports. 2. Breast Diseases—diagnosis—Case Reports. 3. Ultrasonography, Mammary—Case
   Reports. WP 815 H346p 2008]
   RG493.5.R33H42 2008
   618.1′907572—dc22
                                                                                                              2007025627

Important note: Medical knowledge is ever-changing. As new research and clinical experience broaden our knowledge, changes in treatment and drug therapy may be required. The authors and editors of the material herein have consulted sources believed to be reliable in their efforts to provide information that is complete and in accord with the standards accepted at the time of publication. However, in view of the possibility of human error by the authors, editors, or publisher of the work herein or changes in medical knowledge, neither the authors, editors, or publisher, nor any other party who has been involved in the preparation of this work, warrants that the information contained herein is in every respect accurate or complete, and they are not responsible for any errors or omissions or for the results obtained from use of such information. Readers are encouraged to confirm the information contained herein with other sources. For example, readers are advised to check the product information sheet included in the package of each drug they plan to administer to be certain that the information contained in this publication is accurate and that changes have not been made in the recommended dose or in the contraindications for administration. This recommendation is of particular importance in connection with new or infrequently used drugs.

Some of the product names, patents, and registered designs referred to in this book are in fact registered trademarks or proprietary names even though specific reference to this fact is not always made in the text. Therefore, the appearance of a name without designation as proprietary is not to be construed as a representation by the publisher that it is in the public domain.

Printed in the United States

5 4 3 2 1

The Americas ISBN: 978-1-58890-620-5
Rest of World ISBN: 978-3-13-148041-5

This book is dedicated to my parents, Ben and Doris Hashimoto:
The older I become, the more I realize how much I owe you.

Contents

Preface xi

Acknowledgments xiii

1 Historical Review 1

2 Physics of Digital Mammography 4

3 Digital Mammographic Equipment 9
   Lloyd Kreuzer, Ph.D.

4 Normal Anatomy 14

5 Digital Mammographic Appearance of Benign and Malignant Calcifications 19

Cases

5–1	Skin calcifications	Benign	24
5–2	Skin calcifications	Benign	25
5–3	Skin calcifications	Benign	27
5–4	Deodorant	Benign	28
5–5	Milk of calcium	Benign	29
5–6	Milk of calcium	Benign	30
5–7	Vascular calcifications	Benign	31
5–8	Vascular calcifications	Benign	32
5–9	Coarse/popcorn calcifications	Fibroadenoma	33
5–10	Dystrophic calcifications	Fibroadenoma	34
5–11	Dystrophic calcifications	Benign	35
5–12	Dystrophic calcifications	Scar	37
5–13	Dystrophic calcifications	Benign	38
5–14	Dystrophic calcifications	Scar	39
5–15	Eggshell calcifications	Cyst	41
5–16	Round calcifications	Fat necrosis	42
5–17	Round calcifications	Fat necrosis	43
5–18	Punctate calcifications	Sclerosing adenosis	45
5–19	Round calcifications	Calcifications in lobules	46
5–20	Punctate calcifications	Calcifications in lobules	48
5–21	Large rodlike calcifications	Plasma cell mastitis	49
5–22	Punctate calcifications	Calcifications in lobules	51

5–23 Punctate calcifications   Sclerosing adenosis 52
5–24 Punctate calcifications   Calcifications in lobules 53
5–25 Punctate calcifications   Fibrocystic changes 54
5–26 Punctate calcifications   Fibrocystic changes 55
5–27 Punctate calcifications   Atypical ductal hyperplasia............................. 56
5–28 Punctate calcifications   Invasive ductal carcinoma.............................. 57
5–29 Punctate calcifications   Invasive ductal carcinoma.............................. 58
5–30 Amorphous/indistinct calcifications Atypical ductal hyperplasia............................. 59
5–31 Amorphous/indistinct calcifications Ductal carcinoma in situ 60
5–32 Amorphous/indistinct calcifications Ductal carcinoma in situ 62
5–33 Amorphous/indistinct calcifications Ductal carcinoma in situ 64
5–34 Coarse heterogeneous calcifications Fat necrosis 65
5–35 Coarse heterogeneous calcifications Fibrocystic changes 66
5–36 Coarse heterogeneous calcifications Fibroadenoma... 67
5–37 Coarse heterogeneous calcifications Sclerotic papilloma...................................... 68
5–38 Coarse heterogeneous calcifications Ductal carcinoma in situ 69
5–39 Fine pleomorphic calcifications   Fibrocystic changes 70
5–40 Fine pleomorphic calcifications   Fibrocystic changes 71
5–41 Fine pleomorphic calcifications   Fibrocystic changes 72
5–42 Fine pleomorphic calcifications   Atypical ductal hyperplasia............................. 73
5–43 Fine pleomorphic calcifications   Atypical ductal hyperplasia............................. 74
5–44 Fine pleomorphic calcifications   Atypical ductal hyperplasia............................. 76
5–45 Fine pleomorphic calcifications   Ductal carcinoma in situ 77
5–46 Fine pleomorphic calcifications   Ductal carcinoma in situ 78
5–47 Fine pleomorphic calcifications   Ductal carcinoma in situ 79
5–48 Fine pleomorphic calcifications   Ductal carcinoma in situ 80
5–49 Fine pleomorphic calcifications   Ductal carcinoma in situ 82
5–50 Fine pleomorphic calcifications   Ductal carcinoma in situ 83
5–51 Fine pleomorphic calcifications   Ductal carcinoma in situ 84
5–52 Fine pleomorphic calcifications   Infiltrating ductal and ductal carcinoma in situ 85
5–53 Fine linear/branching calcifications Ductal carcinoma in situ 87
5–54 Fine linear/branching calcifications Infiltrating ductal carcinoma 88

6   Digital Mammographic Characteristics of Masses 90

Cases

6–1   Circumscribed mass   Hamartoma... 94
6–2   Circumscribed mass   Lymph node.. 95
6–3   Circumscribed mass   Oil cyst 97
6–4   Circumscribed mass   Pacemaker 99
6–5   Circumscribed mass   Simple cyst 100
6–6   Circumscribed mass   Simple cyst 102
6–7   Circumscribed mass   Simple cyst 104
6–8   Circumscribed mass   Complex cyst... 106
6–9   Circumscribed mass   Simple cyst 108
6–10 Circumscribed mass   Apocrine metaplasia 110
6–11 Circumscribed mass   Fibroadenoma... 112
6–12 Circumscribed mass   Fibroadenoma... 114
6–13 Circumscribed mass   Pseudoangiomatous stromal hyperplasia 116
6–14 Circumscribed mass   Invasive ductal carcinoma.............................. 118
6–15 Circumscribed mass   Invasive ductal carcinoma.............................. 120
6–16 Circumscribed mass   Metaplastic carcinoma 122
6–17 Circumscribed mass   Invasive papillary carcinoma........................... 124
6–18 Circumscribed mass   Intracystic papillary carcinoma 126
6–19 Irregular mass   Fibroadenoma... 128
6–20 Irregular mass   Ductal carcinoma in situ 130
6–21 Irregular mass   Infiltrating ductal carcinoma 131

6–22 Irregular mass   Infiltrating ductal carcinoma 133
6–23 Irregular mass   Infiltrating ductal carcinoma 135
6–24 Irregular mass   Infiltrating ductal carcinoma 137
6–25 Irregular mass   Infiltrating ductal carcinoma 139
6–26 Circumscribed mass   Invasive papillary carcinoma. 141
6–27 Irregular mass   Inflammatory carcinoma 143
6–28 Irregular mass   Inflammatory carcinoma 145

7 Digital Mammographic Technique for Mammographic Asymmetries 148

Cases
7–1   Focal Asymmetry   Fibroadenoma. 154
7–2   Focal Asymmetry   Radial scar 156
7–3   Focal Asymmetry   Infiltrating ductal carcinoma 158
7–4   Focal Asymmetry   Infiltrating ductal carcinoma 160
7–5   Focal Asymmetry   Infiltrating ductal carcinoma 162
7–6   Focal Asymmetry   Infiltrating ductal carcinoma 164
7–7   Focal Asymmetry   Infiltrating ductal carcinoma 166
7–8   Focal Asymmetry   Invasive lobular carcinoma 168
7–9   Focal Asymmetry   Invasive lobular carcinoma 170
7–10 Global Asymmetry   Invasive lobular carcinoma 171
7–11 Global Asymmetry   Infiltrating ductal carcinoma 173

8 Digital Mammographic Characteristics of Architectural Distortion 176

Cases
8–1   Peripheral architectural distortion   Scar. 178
8–2   Peripheral architectural distortion   Radial scar 179
8–3   Subareolar architectural distortion   Infiltrating ductal carcinoma 181
8–4   Subareolar architectural distortion   Invasive ductal carcinoma. 183
8–5   Peripheral architectural distortion   Infiltrating ductal carcinoma 185
8 6   Central architectural distortion   Infiltrating ductal carcinoma 187
8–7   Peripheral architectural distortion   Infiltrating ductal carcinoma 189
8–8   Peripheral architectural distortion   Invasive lobular carcinoma 191
8–9   Central architectural distortion   Infiltrating ductal carcinoma 192
8–10 Central architectural distortion   Radial scar 194

Index 197

Preface

Facing a world with multiple breast imaging techniques, radiologists must now learn how to optimally apply these modalities in the work-up of breast cancer. This book is targeted for breast imagers who are interested in understanding the value of digital mammography within this increasing complex diagnostic armamentarium. Although there is growing interest in the use of other imaging modalities for screening subgroups of women, mammography is still the foundation of general population screening for breast cancer. Therefore, this book is written from the point of view in which digital mammography is the primary screening tool. Like film-screen mammography, digital mammography uses X-rays and is a composite image of the whole breast. However, unlike film-screen mammography, digital mammography's flexibility in acquisition and display has reduced some of the limitations of film-screen technique, particularly in premenopausal women and those with higher fibroglandular composition.

This book addresses some of the clinical uncertainty concerning the indirect mammographic signs of malignancy. In the days when mammography was the only tool, imagers did not have to worry about mammographically occult cancers. However, currently—with increasing use of sonography and magnetic resonance imaging—radiologists have become uncomfortable about what to do when faced with "soft signs" of breast cancer. In traditional mammography books, subtle findings such as asymmetry or one-view architectural distortion are either classified as an obvious mass or are assumed to be normal overlap of glandular tissue. How does one distinguish between these two conclusions? This book analyzes digital mammographic techniques that one may use to solve this problem. The tables associating digital mammographic findings with American College of Radiology assessment categories are devised to create a structure for this problem-solving approach. These tables are not meant to be legal guidelines or documents. These tables are designed to provide an organizational approach to the study of digital mammographic findings that will hopefully aid one in reaching a reasonable conclusion or assessment.

This book is also meant for the radiologist, resident, or technologist who is facing the challenge of organizing a digital mammographic imaging center. This text is meant to be a practical book that provides information about digital mammographic physics and equipment which will allow one to intelligently compare technologies and systems. As an imager that has been involved with digital equipment evaluation and purchase for 20 years, I have found many factors in the evolution of digital mammography that are common to those that I have experienced with other digital imaging conversions. Some of the major challenges include: large expense; rapidly changing technology, and inconsistent connectivity; and finally, need for strong information technology support.

The initial conversion cost to digital mammographic imaging is relatively expensive due to the cost of digital mammography hardware, software, and storage. Even if one's center is completely converted to digital mammography, one will need to develop methods to incorporate review of analog images either from other institutions or from one's own previous exams. The conversion may involve other internal information systems in the development of new schemes to transfer digital exams to other institutions.

Since digital mammography technology is relatively new, there is rapid increase in the number of systems available, and the extant products are rapidly improving. Imagers investing in digital mammography are faced with the challenge of avoiding equipment that will be quickly out-of-date. In addition, industry standardization is also relatively new, and connectivity between vendors is not well-established. Radiologists developing a breast imaging center face frustration in trying to design a customized framework consisting of multiple vendors. Even if the mammographic images can be transferred from an acquisition station to a different vendor workstation, the images may not be easily interpreted since the post-processing of the mammograms may be proprietary and therefore not transferable.

Finally, the breast imager who plans for a digital environment is also challenged with developing a new technical support system. Besides being familiar with hardware, the support group needs to understand informational transfer issues. Development of a strong support team is crucial for the success of digital mammography.

With the significant cost and difficulties faced by radiologists and administrators in developing a digital mammographic center, why would anyone do it? The simplistic answer is to reduce the cost of film. However, as stated earlier, the cost of converting to digital mammography is expensive: generally greater than the price of film alone. Some of the expense can be saved in improved technologist efficiency. Studies have shown that digital mammography, like other digital techniques, does improve technologist efficiency. Therefore, when replacing analog with digital mammographic units, most centers are able to greatly reduce the number of total mammographic acquisition stations.

Although the relative efficiency of digital mammography associated with reduction in film costs commonly is the basis for conversion to digital mammography, these advantages do not account for the great clinical advantages of digital mammography. A global view of radiology would suggest that digital mammography is the future form of mammography. Virtually all other imaging modalities are being converted to purely digital storage and transfer, and the digital trend in mammography is inevitable. Technical advantages of digital mammography are described in the following chapters. However, the improved flexibility in image display and transfer are some of its strongest features.

In conclusion, although there are increasing imaging modalities that may be used to evaluate breast disease, mammography will continue to play a key role in detecting breast cancer. To be an effective imager, the radiologist should become familiar with digital mammography and understand its role within the increasing complex structure of breast imaging techniques.

Acknowledgments

I have been lucky to have found a professional home at Virginia Mason Medical Center for over 20 years. One of the major reasons that I have enjoyed breast imaging is the people who surround me. They have always valued clinical research to improve patient care. In particular, I am grateful to the clinical support and expertise of my fellow breast radiologists, including Drs. Stephen Adler, "Butch" Hartzog, Dawna Kramer, Marie Lee, Matthew McCormick, Gail Morgan, and Alexi Phinney. They are always ready to share interesting images, discuss difficult clinical problems, and provide technical advice. The rest of the radiologist group at Virginia Mason has also been extremely clinically supportive. I am indebted for the advice and information on breast magnetic resonance imaging from Drs. Felicia Cummings, Lucy Glenn, Larry Holder, and Marc Lacrampe. I also especially appreciate the administrative support from my Department Chief, Dr. Lucy Glenn and Administrative Director, Jim Sapienza.

I want to thank the technical staff in the Virginia Mason Breast Center for their hard work and dedication: they inspire me every day. As in many departments, the satisfaction of patients is due to the conscientious work of the medical assistants and mammographers: Dyan Blaze, Amy Chu, Pat Dennis, Elena Ermolenko, Mary Ann Fernandez, Jaime Heinrichs, Mary Anne Madsen, Emma Orejudos, Diana Pearsall, Kimberly Peery, Karen Waalkes, Tess Wilcynski, Krystyna Wojtulewicz, Susanne Ziegler, and manager Sharon Hemphill. The quality of the breast ultrasound images is due to the contributions of sonographers: Irina Askerova, Stacy Buck, Chris Chapman, Valerie Holland, Nancy Honssinger, Ashliegh Joyce, Ashley Little, Suzy Murray Dirks, Lynette Passey, Ann Polin, Gisele Sodell, Emily Whiting, Jackie Wyngaard, and manager Shannon Boswell.

I have been indebted to our image management team who cheerfully and rapidly obtain images archived from previous years: Scott Borman, Jon Komatsu, Alice Wirth, Linda O'Connell, Rosalinda Argonza, Tino Ativalu, Agnes Celmar, Jonathan Fernandez, Tracy Guster, Henock Kidane, Martin Medina, James Reyes, Kathy Salzinger, Grace Viloria.

I also appreciate the assistance of Anhaita Jamula and Joanne VanderDoes in processing and reviewing my images and organizing my research efforts, and a special thanks to Jean Nelson for administrative help. A strong information systems team is a key element for digital imaging success, and I particularly thank our Radiology Applications Support Team: Courtney Allen, Scott Hamilton, Jerry Bullock and Michelle Ranous for their expertise. Finally although all the images are digital, I have depended upon the special talents of the Virginia Mason Medical Photography Department for digital processing asssistance: Terrance King, Bob Riedinger and Taylor Ubben. I want to relay a special thanks to Morris Ferensen who has been an invaluable advisor about image processing. I am also blessed to know a talented artist, Joanne Clifford, who created the schematic drawings.

At Thieme Publishers, I have been lucky to work with Timothy Hiscock who has provided guidance in developing and completing this project. I am particularly indebted to him for his professional literary support. Thieme editorial assistants David Price and Joycelyn Reed have patiently reviewed the manuscript and images and provided valuable feedback.

Finally, I would not have completed this book without the encouragement of my family: parents Doris and Ben, sister Claire, brothers Dean and Gary, husband Vincent, and children Ben, Dean, and Elissa. The joy I have at work is a reflection of their love.

1 Historical Review

From 1960 to 1990, multiple large prospective randomized trials were performed to test if screen-film mammography reduced female mortality. The most commonly reviewed trials include the following (starting dates of the trials are in parentheses): the Health Insurance Plan (HIP) of New York (1963); the Edinburgh trial (1979); two Canadian trials—National Breast Screening Study (NBSS) 1 and 2 (both 1980); and four Swedish trials—Swedish Two County (1977), Malmö (1976), Stockholm (1981), and Gothenburg (1982). The HIP, Swedish Two County, Malmö, and Edinburgh trials all showed a statistically significant reduction in mortality (between 19% and 32%) in screened women compared with women who were not mammographically screened. The Stockholm and Gothenburg trials showed that there was 20 to 23% lower mortality in the screened populations, but these reductions were not statistically significant.[1,2] The Canadian studies resulted in the worst performance for screening mammography. The Canadian NBSS-2, which included women 50 to 59 years of age, found only a 2% mortality reduction in the screened group after 13 years of follow-up, and the NBSS-1, which studied women ages 40 to 49, reported 7% more breast cancer deaths after 16 years.[1–3]

Proof of mortality reduction requires large numbers of participants. To obtain statistical significance, researchers have retrospectively combined the data from the previously described screening trials. A meta-analysis of all of these major trials plus four other case-controlled studies in 1995 found that there was a statistically significant (26%) reduction in mortality for women ages 50 to 74. No significant reduction in breast cancer mortality was identified in women ages 40 to 49.[4] The results of this study reflected the general results of previous meta-analyses and supported further analysis of the data from younger screened women. Meta-analysis of the randomized controlled trials in 1997 found that there was a statistically significant reduction in mortality for women ages 40 to 74. Specifically, the reduction for women ages 40 to 49 was 18%; for women ages 50 to74, it was 24%. When only data from the Swedish trials were combined, this study found that the mortality reduction for women ages 40 to 49 was 29%.[5] Since that time, other meta-analyses have reported similar statistically significant levels in mortality reduction for women ages 40 to 74.[6,7]

As digital mammographic machines matured, trials were performed on these units to discover if digital mammography was an effective screening tool. Early trials were performed primarily to obtain U.S. Food and Drug Administration (FDA) approval for specific digital mammography devices. Because screen-film mammography had already had a long history of research validation, the main goal of these trials was to demonstrate that digital mammography was substantially equivalent to screen-film technology. Hendrick led a multinstitutional trial testing the General Electric Senographe 2000D (GE Healthcare, formerly General Electric Medical Systems, Chalfont St. Giles, United Kingdom) involving 625 women who had both digital and screen-film mammograms. He reported that the sensitivity for digital mammography was 55% versus 53% for screen film mammography, and the specificity for digital was 68% compared with 70% for screen-film mammography. Although these differences were not statistically significant, digital mammography was associated with a 2% lower recall rate, which was statistically significant.[8]

Pisano led the multinstitutional trial to test the Fischer SenoScan (Fischer Imaging Corp., Denver, Colorado). This study involved a review of digital and screen-film mammograms from 676 women. The sensitivity of digital mammography was 66% compared with 74% for screen-film; the specificities were 67% for digital and 60% for screen-film mammography. These differences were not statistically significant.[8,9]

To obtain greater statistical power, larger prospective randomized trials have been performed to compare the accuracy of screen-film mammography and digital mammography. Starting in 1998, researchers at the University of Colorado and the University of Massachusetts enrolled 4489 women who had 6736 pairs of screen-film and digital mammogram examinations. This trial, which was supported by the U.S. Department of Defense, reported that of 42 total cancers, 33 were detected with screen-film and 25 with digital mammography. There was no significant difference in the sensitivities between digital (54%) and screen-film (66%) mammography. The free-response receiver operating characteristic curve for digital mammography had a slightly smaller area under the curve (0.74) compared with screen-film (0.80), but this difference was not statistically significant. However, the investigators did find that the difference in the recall rate for digital mammography (11.8%) was statistically significantly lower compared with screen-film mammography (14.9%).[8,10,11]

Two prospective trials, Oslo I and II, were performed in Norway in 2000 and 2001. The earlier Oslo I trial involved 3683 women who had both screen-film and digital mammography. Of a total 31 cancers, the research mammographers found 23 cancers with digital mammography and 28 malignancies by screen-film mammography. The cancer detection rate for digital mammography was 62%, 76% for screen-film. This difference was not statistically significant. Contrary to previous studies, these investigators had a higher recall rate with digital (4.6%) compared with screen-film (3.5%) mammography.[12] Two-year follow-up continued to demonstrate no significant difference in these findings.[13]

In the Oslo II trial, the research group randomized 25,263 women for either screen-film mammography or digital mammography. In the 6,997 women who had digital mammography, 41 cancers were identified, for a detection rate of 0.59%. This digital detection rate was better than the detection rate of screen-film mammography: 73 cancers were identified in 17,911 women with screen-film mammography, for a detection rate of 0.41%. This difference did not reach statistical significance ($p = .06$). Similar to the Oslo I trial, this trial found that the recall rate for digital mammography was significantly higher (3.8%) compared with screen-film mammography (2.5%) in women ages 50 to 69 years ($p < .05$).[14]

The National Cancer Institute funded the American College of Radiology Imaging Network (ACRIN), a cooperative group established to examine the efficacy of digital mammography. This group developed the Digital Mammographic Imaging Screening Trial (DMIST) to compare the accuracy of digital to screen-film mammography for screening asymptomatic women.[15] Starting in 2001, 33 U.S. and Canadian sites enrolled 49,528 women to undergo both digital and screen-film mammography. The sensitivities of digital and screen-film mammography were not significantly different for the entire population. The sensitivity and specificity of digital mammography were 70% and 92%, respectively, versus 66 and 92%, respectively, for screen-film mammography. The authors attributed the relatively low sensitivities to the longer clinical patient follow-up (455 days compared with the 365-day follow-up in previous studies).[16]

Although the diagnostic sensitivity of digital and screen-film was not statistically different for the entire population, the study demonstrated that digital mammography was significantly more accurate than screen-film mammography among three female groups: women with heterogeneously dense or extremely dense breasts, women under the age of 50 years, and in premenopausal or perimenopausal women. Whereas, for these three groups, the sensitivities of digital mammography ranged from 70 to 80%, the sensitivities of screen-film were only 50 to 55%. The researchers suggested that the relative success of digital mammography in these groups was due to the mammographer's ability to manipulate the digital image contrast and identify subtle lesions.[16]

The findings that digital mammography is more accurate than screen-film in those with relatively dense breasts and in younger women are important potential advantages of the digital technique. Although screen-film mammography has been accepted as an effective method to screen for breast cancer, closer evaluation of the screen-film technique has shown that both breast fibroglandular composition and age affect the accuracy of this test. Sensitivity of screen-film mammography is highest in women with completely fatty breasts (sensitivity 88%, specificity 97%) compared with women with extremely dense breasts (sensitivity 62%, specificity 90%). Furthermore, screen-film mammography performs better in older women compared with younger women. Sensitivity for women ages 80 to 89 is 86% compared with 66% for women ages 40 to 49.[17]

Studies recording the parenchymal composition categories described by the Breast Imaging Reporting and Data System (BI-RADS) have reported that ~45% of screening mammograms are classified as heterogeneously dense or extremely dense.[10,18] Because the sensitivity and specificity of screen-film mammography decrease with increasing fibroglandular composition, digital mammography may potentially benefit almost half of all screening women. Furthermore, in women under the age of 50, the relative strength of digital mammography is complementary to a known weakness in screen-film mammography. The application of digital mammography for younger women and women with relatively dense breasts may improve in breast cancer screening for these groups.

In summary, prospective randomized trials comparing digital mammography with screen-film have found that the performance of digital mammography for all women 40 years and older is similar to screen-film mammography. However, the DMIST study found that digital mammography was superior to screen-film for breast cancer screening in women who were premenopausal or perimenopausal, were 50 years of age or younger, or had heterogeneous or extremely dense breasts. These categories are a known weakness of screen-film mammography, so these applications alone would make digital mammography a useful breast imaging technique. Because the availability of digital screening is still extremely limited,[19] in facilities that have both screen-film and digital techniques, individualizing the technique according to age, menopausal status, and, if available, breast composition category would be a method to optimize screening imaging.[20]

References

1. Smith RA, D'Orsi CJ. Screening for breast cancer. In: Harris JR, Mippman ME, Morrow M, Osborne CK., eds. Diseases of the Breast. Philadelphia: Lippincott Williams & Wilkins; 2004:103–130
2. Feig SA. Screening results, controversies, and guidelines. In: Bassett LW, Jackson VP, Fu KL, Fu YS, eds. Diagnosis of Diseases of the Breast. 2nd ed. Philadelphia: Elsevier, Saunders; 2005:371–387
3. Miller AB, To T, Baines CJ, Wall C. The Canadian National Breast Screening Study-1: breast cancer mortality after 11 to 16 years of follow-up. Ann Intern Med 2002;137:305–312
4. Kerlikowske K, Grady D, Rubin SM, Sandrock C, Ernster VL. Efficacy of screening mammography: a meta-analysis. JAMA 1995;273:149–154

5. Hendrick RE, Smith RA, Rutledge JH, Smart CR. Benefit of screening mammography in women aged 40–49: a new meta-analysis of randomized controlled trials [abstract]. J Natl Cancer Inst Monogr 1997;22:87–92

6. Humphrey LL, Helfand M, Chan BKS, Woolf SH. Breast cancer screening: a summary of the evidence for the U.S. Preventive Services Task Force. Ann Intern Med 2002;137:347–360

7. Fletcher SW, Elmore JG. Mammographic screening for breast cancer. N Engl J Med 2003;348:1672–1680

8. Pisano ED. Digital mammography trials. In: Pisano ED, Yaffe MJ, Kuzmiak CM, eds. Digital Mammography. Philadelphia: Lippincott Williams & Wilkins; 2003:27–32

9. Cole E, Pisano ED, Brown M, et al. Diagnostic accuracy of Fischer SenoScan digital mammography versus screen-film mammography in a diagnostic mammography population. Acad Radiol 2004;11:879–886

10. Lewin JM, Hendrick RE, D'Orsi CJ, et al. Comparison of full-field digital mammography with screen-film mammography for cancer detection: results of 4945 paired examinations. Radiology 2001;218:873–880

11. Lewin JM, D'Orsi CJ, Hendrick RE, et al. Clinical comparison of full-field digital mammography and screen-film mammography for detection of breast cancer. AJR Am J Roentgenol 2002;179:671–677

12. Skaane P, Young K, Skjennald A. Population-based mammography screening: comparison of screen-film and full-field digital mammography with soft copy reading—Oslo I study. Radiology 2003;229:877–884

13. Skaane P, Skjennald A, Young K, et al. Follow-up and final results of the Oslo I study comparing screen-film mammography and full-field digital mammography with soft-copy reading. Acta Radiol 2005;46:679–689

14. Skaane P, Skjennald A. Screen-film mammography versus full-field digital mammography with soft-copy reading: randomized trial in a population-based screening program—the Oslo II study. Radiology 2004;232:197–204

15. Pisano ED, Gatsonis CA, Yaffe MJ, et al. American College of Radiology Imaging Network Digital Mammographic Imaging Screening Trial: objectives and methodology. Radiology 2005;236:404–412

16. Pisano ED, Gatsonis C, Hendrick RE, et al. Diagnostic performance of digital versus film mammography for breast-cancer screening. N Engl J Med 2005;353:1773–1783

17. Carney PA, Miglioretti DL, Yankaskas BC, et al. Individual and combined effects of age, breast density, and hormone replacement therapy use on the accuracy of screening mammography. Ann Intern Med 2003;138:168–175

18. Venta LA, Hendrick RE, Adler YT, et al. Rates and causes of disagreement in interpretation of full-field digital mammography and film-screen mammography in a diagnostic setting. Am J Roentgenol 2001;176:1241–1248

19. Hendrick RE, Cutter GR, Berns EA, et al. Community-based mammography practice: services, charges, and interpretation methods. Am J Roentgenol 2005;184:433–438

20. Dershaw DD. Status of mammography after the digital mammography imaging screening trial: digital versus film. Breast J 2006;12:99–102

2 Physics of Digital Mammography

A basic understanding of the principles of physics is useful in evaluating equipment and understanding the factors that affect the quality of the digital image. Digital signals are transmitted in multiples of defined equal signals. A common item that displays either analog or digital information is the watch. The second hand of the analog watch sweeps around the dial in a continuous 360-degree motion. One second is not discretely separated from the next. In fact, theoretically, it should be possible to time actions to a tenth or a hundredth of a second. However, practically speaking, the second hand moves too quickly for this type of measurement. When a digital watch displays seconds, the watch presents each second as a discrete whole number. The watch does not show any intervening tenth or hundredth of a second. There is only a change in the number when one whole second has passed. With digital transmission, information is relayed in discrete packets of information.

Digital information is described using the terms pixels and bits or bytes. A pixel is a picture element. A digital image consists of a rectangular matrix of pixels. The size of the digital image is described as the number of horizontal pixels by the number of vertical pixels. Therefore, an image identified as 500 by 300 pixels refers to a rectangular matrix that is 500 pixels wide and 300 pixels high (**Fig. 2–1**). Because mammograms are displayed in various shades of gray, each pixel can potentially display a fixed maximal number of gray shades. The number of shades is described by bits. A bit is defined as 2^X, where

X is the number of bits. So, 8 bits is 256 shades of gray. A 12-bit image has 4096 shades of gray. Finally, 8 bits equals 1 byte. The total size of an image is described as the total number of pixels multiplied by the number of bits per pixel. Therefore, if the previously described image consisting of 500 by 300 pixels had a gray scale consisting of 8 bits, the total number of bits in the image would be 500 × 300 × 8 or 1,200,000 bits or 150,000 bytes. Familiarity with this numerical terminology is important because in digital imaging, these terms are used for a variety of applications: to express the amount of information within a digital mammogram, to describe the resolution of a workstation monitor, and to measure the amount of digital space needed for long-term storage.[1]

■ Image Acquisition Physics

Digital Detector Characteristic Curve Versus Screen-Film

One major difference in the physics of the digital mammography system and a screen-film system is the digital mammographic detector. The digital detector replaces the screen and film components of nondigital or analog mammography machines. The image produced by screen-film mammography is described by the characteristic curve that plots the relationship between film density on the vertical axis

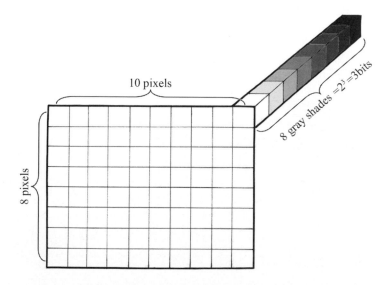

Figure 2–1 Schematic illustrating digital image matrix. The image consists of a matrix of picture elements (pixels). A digital image consists of a rectangular matrix of pixels. The size of the digital image is described by the number of horizontal pixels by the number of vertical pixels. Therefore, this rectangular matrix image is identified as 10 by 8 pixels. Each pixel is associated with a fixed number of gray-scale shades defined by bits (a bit is defined as 2^X, where X is the number of bits). This image has eight shades of gray, or 2^3 or 3 bits. The total size of an image is described as the total number of pixels multiplied by the number of bits per pixel. Therefore, the total size of this image is 10 × 8 × 8 or 640 bits, or 80 bytes.

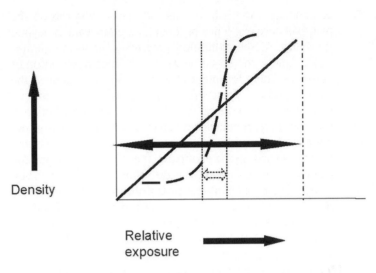

Density

Relative exposure

Figure 2–2 Characteristic curves for digital detectors and film. The relationship between exposure (horizontal axis) and density (vertical axis) is shown by the black dashed curve for film and the solid slanted line for digital detectors. The narrow latitude (*dotted arrow*) of film is contrasted with the wide latitude (*solid black arrow*) for digital detectors.[1]

and the relative exposure on the horizontal axis (**Fig. 2–2**). In order to produce a mammogram that has a wide range of tissue densities, you should use exposures that result in densities that align with the steep part of the curve. This set of densities is the latitude of the film. Screen-film mammography has a relatively narrow latitude. However, digital detectors are created so that there is a linear relationship between density and relative exposure. This relationship produces a wider latitude. The latitude of digital mammography is ~1000:1 compared with 40:1 for screen film mammography. This wider latitude results in a broader range of exposures that will produce an acceptable image.[2,3]

Digital latitude is related to dynamic range or the depth of recorded signal intensity. In a gray-scale image, dynamic range is recorded as a series of gray scale shades. The numerical value of the dynamic range is expressed as bits or 2^x steps of digitalization. The dynamic range required for digital mammographic imaging is related to the number of gray-scale shades that will adequately display the structures that attenuate the most and the fewest x-rays within the breast. The attenuation of x-rays is related to three factors: the energy of the x-ray, the breast thickness, and the breast tissue (fatty vs. fibroglandular).

The following example demonstrates the general method that is used to determine the adequacy of digital mammographic detector dynamic range. In this example, to simplify the problem, you would make the following assumptions: (1) The incident x-ray is a monoenergetic 25 keV (kiloelectronvolt). (2) The breast is uniformly compressed to only 8 cm. (3) Part of this breast is composed of 0% fibroglandular tissue (i.e., almost entirely fat). (4) Part of this breast is composed of 100% fibroglandular tissue (this is extremely dense composition). After the incident x-ray passes through the hypothetical breast, the relative attenuation produced by the fibroglandular composition is calculated, taking into account the breast thickness and the x-ray keV. The calculated factors for this hypothetical mammogram are authentic and displayed in **Table 2–1**.[4]

When you administer 25 keV x-rays to the 8 cm breast, the incident x-ray is attenuated a factor of 57, where the breast composition is 100% fibroglandular, versus a factor of 13, where the breast is 0% fibroglandular. After superficial examination of this situation, you might consider using 7 bit digitalization (128 steps). With 7 bit digitalization, the signal from the 100% fibroglandular composition would be 2 (128/57 = 2.25). This signal would be differentiated from the signal resulting from fatty composition, which would be 10 (128/13 = 9.8). However, if a suspicious mass had an attenuation of 56, then the detector signal would be 128/56, or 2.29. Because the signal would be recorded in whole numbers, the final outgoing signal would be 2—the same apparent number as 100% fibroglandular composition. The signal from the abnormality would not be separable from the fibroglandular tissue. To segregate these signals, you would need ~100 times the original gray-scale steps. If you had a dynamic range that was 100 times the original dynamic range, the lesion would produce a signal of 229, and the surrounding fibroglandular tissue would produce a signal of 225. Therefore, increasing the dynamic range separates the fibroglandular tissue signal from the suspicious mass. To obtain this better signal separation, in this hypothetical example, you would need a minimum of 57 (maximum factor) × 100, or 5700, steps. Therefore, you would need ~13 bits (8192 steps) of digitalization. Twelve bits (4096 steps) would not be adequate in this example. Currently, digital mammography detectors have dynamic ranges between 12 and 14 bits[4] (**Table 2–1**).

Table 2–1 Attenuation of Incident 25 keV X-rays

Attenuating Influences	Breast Thickness	Fibroglandular Tissue (5)		
	8 cm	0%	50%	100%
Factor by which x-rays attenuated		13	27	57

Source: Data from Feig SA, Yaffe MJ. Digital mammography. Radiographics 1998;18:893–901.

Spatial Resolution

The spatial resolution of digital detectors is affected by different factors compared with screen-film technology. Screen-film technology is superior in spatial resolution. With optimal imaging, screen-film images exhibit 20 line pairs per millimeter (20 lp/mm). This resolution is equivalent to pixels that are 25 µm apart. Digital detectors generally have a resolution of ~5 to 10 lp/mm, or pixels ~50 to 100 µm apart.[5]

The resolution of the detector is generally determined by the size of the del. The del is the smallest detector element. Digital detectors are usually composed of numerous dels. For example, in the thallium-activated cesium iodide (CsI (Tl)) phosphor flat-panel detector, the del consists of the photodiode and the thin film transistor. In the computed radiography system, the del is determined by the size of the laser beam and the distance between the sampled measurements.[4]

The resolution of the final digital image is described by the modulation transfer function (MTF). In both screen-film and digital mammography, the image is affected by multiple processes such as the del, the focal spot size, the magnification, and the spread of signal within the detector. The MTF is a method to measure the effect of multiple factors on the resolution of the image.[6-10] The general intuitive principle of the effect of multiple processes on the MTF has been clearly described by Christensen and colleagues in their classic radiology physics book.[11] If MTF represents a change or modulation in the amount or intensity of information, assume you have a can of thick oil, and the oil represents information. If you pour the oil from the can into a glass container, some of the oil will stick to the original can. Therefore, there will be less oil, or information, in the glass container compared with the original can. The resulting oil, or information, in the glass container has been changed or modulated. You can identify the amount of modulation or change by measuring the oil in the glass container and comparing this volume to the original amount in the can. In this analogy, the MTF would be described using this equation:

$$MTF = information_{out}/information_{in}$$

The analogy demonstrates that when information is modulated or changed, the total amount of information never increases. At best, the total information stays the same; that is, the MTF equals 1. However, generally, the total information is reduced; in this case, the MTF is less than 1.[11]

The actual physics of the MTF graph is more complex and beyond the scope of this text. However, the general principle is that the information is changed or modulated as it proceeds through a radiographic system. This modification or change in information is compared with increasing spatial frequency. Another analogy that describes the MTF graph is the following: There is an outdoor painting exhibition. A painting team consists of two players and a basket of paintballs. The paintballs are flexible so that they will slide through tight spaces. The first player grabs a paint-

ball and gives the ball to a second player, who throws the paintball between fence posts to hit a white canvas beyond the fence. As the exhibition progresses, only one parameter changes: the space between the fence posts becomes narrower. There is a point at which the space between the fence posts is too narrow for the paintballs to pass, so that no paint will land on the canvas. The decreasing space between the fence posts is equivalent to increasing line pairs, improving spatial resolution, or increasing frequency. If you assume that the volume in the paintball is the information in and the paint volume on the canvas is the information out, then you can graph the paint volume against the increasing frequency (**Fig. 2–3**). In this example, the MTF is measuring the efforts of the entire system: the players, the paintballs, the fence, and canvas relationships. If you change any of the factors, such as decreasing the size of the paintballs or bringing the fence closer to the canvas, then the MTF will change.

When comparing MTFs of various digital mammographic machines, systems that exhibit better preservation of resolution exhibit higher MTF levels per spatial frequency (**Fig. 2–3**). Besides being useful in comparing different digital mammographic systems, MTF curves are an important factor to check as part of the quality control procedure because they will indicate if there is a breakdown in the processes surrounding digital imaging production and display.[6-10]

Noise

In a digital mammographic detector, there are four types of noise: quantum, fixed electronic, secondary signal, and indirect secondary quanta. Both screen-film and digital mammographic detectors are subject to random fluctuation of x-ray quanta, or quantum mottle. This fluctuation is

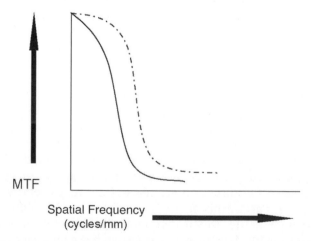

Figure 2–3 Modulation transfer function (MTF). The curve exhibits the MTF on the vertical axis and spatial frequency (cycles/mm) on the horizontal axis. Hypothetical MTFs for two different radiographic systems are illustrated. The MTF for the system with the dotted curve demonstrates less reduction in resolution compared with the system with the solid curve.

due to the random spatial variation of x-rays absorbed by the detector. If more x-rays are used to produce the image, then the effect of quantum mottle would be reduced. In a digital mammographic exam, the reduction in quantum mottle may be accomplished by increasing the signal-to-noise ratio (SNR). To improve SNR, you would apply the appropriate x-ray exposure and have a detector with optimum quantum interaction efficiency. Higher quantum interaction efficiency corresponds to a higher fraction of x-rays that the detector converts into digital signals.[12]

Because of the rigid matrix of their structures, digital detectors generate a fixed electronic structural noise. This structural noise pattern is removed by flat fielding correction. This technical correction is an important part of the digital mammographic quality control process.[12,13]

The third type of noise produced by digital detectors is secondary signal. When the x-ray strikes a phosphor crystal, one or more light quanta may be produced. The number of light quanta produced follows a statistical distribution that is related either to the percent of x-ray energy converted to light or to the presence of multiple x-ray energies present within the emitted beam. This fluctuation in light quanta results in secondary signal noise.[12,13]

Finally, indirect secondary noise may be present in detectors that use a multistep process in converting x-rays to digital information. In detectors that convert the x-ray to light before changing the light into an electrical signal, there will be a fluctuation in the production of light quanta that are detected and captured for the final conversion. If the capture and conversion of light are inefficient, then this indirect noise may become significant.[12]

Artifacts

Digital mammography, like screen-film technique, may produce artifacts. Digital artifacts include flat fielding artifacts, stitching, dead pixels, and scanning artifacts. Flat fielding nonuniformity was discussed earlier. The individual elements of the detector matrix may drift in sensitivity to different intensities, so regular testing and recalibration are necessary to correct this problem. Stitching results from gaps between the edges of the individual detector elements. Because digital detectors are generally formed

from multiple small detector components, inactivation or damage to one or more of these elements will produce irregularities in the digital image. Finally, any malfunction in a mechanical component of a detector will produce artifacts in the image. If the laser beam reader movement becomes irregular or there is misalignment between the x-ray beam and the slot collimator, there will be problems with the digital image.[9,12,14]

■ Digital Image Display

Soft Copy

Digital mammographic images may be transferred and interpreted on high-resolution monitors. These monitors generally have a matrix that is 2.0 by 2.5 Kpixels, or 5.0 Mpixels in size.[5] There should be minimum ambient light (i.e., < 5 lux). Even if a center converts completely to full-field digital mammography, the reading area should be designed to accommodate hard copy films from earlier years or other institutions. This design generally involved a set of digital workstation monitors and either stationary view boxes or, preferably, a multiviewer with high-luminance view boxes. The interpretive workstation monitors should be placed so there is minimum glare reflecting from one set of monitors to the other. The American College of Radiology Imaging Network's Digital Mammography Imaging Screening Trial (DMIST) recommended that incident light on the monitor surface not exceed 10 lux.[10] One solution is to have the monitors at right angles to the view boxes to minimize this reflection.[2]

■ Digital Image Storage

The storage for full-field digital mammography is determined by the size of each image. The size of the image is equal to the length in pixels multiplied by the width in pixels by the number of intensity levels or shades of gray. Most systems digitize the signal into 2^{12} or 2^{14} intensity levels, or 12 or 14 bits within each pixel. Depending on the image size, a four-view screening mammographic examination requires between 30 and 200 MB (megabytes) of computer storage space[2] (see Chapter 3).

References

1. James JJ. The current status of digital mammography. Clin Radiol 2004;59:1–10
2. Mahesh M. AAPM/RSNA Physics tutorial for residents: digital mammography: an overview. Radiographics 2004;24:1747–1760
3. Feig SA, Yaffe MJ. Digital mammography. Radiographics 1998;18:893–901
4. Yaffe MJ. Physics of digital mammography. In: Pisano ED, Yaffe MJ, Kuzmiak CM, eds. Digital Mammography. Philadelphia: Lippincott Williams & Wilkins; 2003:4–14
5. Ikeda DM. Mammographic acquisition: screen-film and digital mammography, computer-aided detection, and the mammography quality standards act. In: Breast Imaging: The Requisites. Philadelphia: Elsevier Mosby; 2004:1–23
6. Monnin P, Gutierrez D, Bulling S, Lepori D, Valley JF, Verdun FR. A comparison of the performance of modern screen-film and digital mammography systems. Phys Med Biol 2005;50:2617–2631
7. Marshall NW. A comparison between objective and subjective image quality measurements for a full field digital mammography system. Phys Med Biol 2006;51:2441–2463
8. Carton A-K, Vandenbroucke D, Struye L, et al. Validation of MTF measurement for digital mammography quality control. Med Phys 2005;32:1684–1695

9. Bloomquist AK, Yaffe MJ, Pisano ED, et al. Quality control for digital mammography in the ACRIN DMIST trial: part I. Med Phys 2006;33:719–736

10. Yaffe MJ, Bloomquist AK, Mawdsley GE, et al. Quality control for digital mammography: part II. Recommendations from the ACRIN DMIST trial. Med Phys 2006;33:737–752

11. Christensen EF, Curry TS, Dowdey JF, eds. Geometry of the radiographic image. In: An Introduction to the Physics of Diagnostic Radiology. Philadelphia: Lea & Febiger; 1978: 152–184

12. Haus AG, Yaffe MJ. Screen-film and digital mammography image quality and radiation dose considerations. Radiol Clin North Am 2000;28:871–898

13. Yaffe MJ, Mainprize JG. Detectors for digital mammography. In: Pisano ED, Yaffe MJ, Kuzmiak CM, eds. Digital Mammography. Philadelphia: Lippincott Williams & Wilkins; 2003:15–32

14. Yaffe MJ. Quality control for digital mammography. In: Pisano ED, Yaffe MJ, Kuzmiak CM, eds. Digital Mammography. Philadelphia: Lippincott Williams & Wilkins; 2003:33–42

3 Digital Mammography Equipment

Lloyd Kreuzer, Ph.D.[*]

Mammography technology may be divided into three functions: image acquisition, display, and storage. With screen-film mammography, the image acquisition process starts when the breast is exposed to x-rays. As the x-rays pass through the breast, they are absorbed and scattered within the tissues. The attenuated x-rays pass through a grid, interact with the image receptor, and form a latent image on film. The exposed film is processed by reducing the silver ions in the x-ray film emulsion to metallic silver. The film is then treated with fixer that both removes excess silver and is a preservative. Finally, the film is rinsed to remove fixer.[1] The resulting film is the key medium that is used for both display and later storage.

Image acquisition, display, and archiving are interlinked by screen-film mammography. For example, if the mammogram is suboptimally acquired and is too light, display of the image on a view box will be compromised. There is no screen-film display method that will correct this problem. However, with digital mammography, image acquisition, display, and archival functions involve separate systems. This separation of function is important because in screen-film mammography, any problem with one of the functions affects the quality of the entire process. However, with digital mammography, each process may be optimized independently of the other functions. This separation of function allows digital mammography to take advantage of several technical opportunities. For example, researchers have found that although 4% of digital mammograms are poorly exposed, 100% of the final mammographic displays are adequate as a result of digital postprocessing.[2]

■ Digital Acquisition

There are two types of digital mammography acquisition systems: one based on digital x-ray technology and the other based on computed radiology (CR) technology. Digital x-ray systems convert x-rays directly to a digital image. The conversion occurs essentially instantaneously. CR systems expose a CR plate to x-rays and then "read" the image from the plate by scanning the plate with a laser beam. These systems also generate a digital image, but the image is generated when the plate is read and not at the time of exposure. Digital x-ray systems have the advantage of generating an image instantly after the exposure. This provides rapid feedback to the technician if the image is suboptimal, such as when the patient is poorly positioned. CR systems are typically less expensive than digital x-ray systems.

There are three types of direct digital x-ray systems: (1) those with cesium iodide (CsI) phosphor detector systems, (2) those with selenium, and (3) those with quantum counting detectors. CsI phosphor systems were the first flat-plate mammographic detectors available in the United States. Thallium-activated cesium iodide [CsI (T1)] crystals were developed for digital mammographic systems because these crystals produce better resolution compared with earlier conventional x-ray phosphors. The CsI (T1) crystals form thin columns. The light produced by the crystal passes down the column to the photodiode. Compared with other phosphors, the C_sI (T1) crystals reduce the lateral spread of the light and improve resolution.

Like a multilayer cake, the CsI phosphor detector has three layers (**Fig. 3–1**). The base of this detector is coated with a layer of amorphous silicon. On top of this silicon is a layer of light-sensitive photodiodes. Each photodiode is a tiny square. These photodiodes form a matrix that microscopically looks like a quilt. Each photodiode contains a thin-film transistor switch. Finally, a layer of thallium-activated C_sI (Tl) crystals are deposited on the photodiodes.

The CsI flat panel works in the following manner. When an x-ray strikes a CsI (Tl) crystal, the crystal produces light. The light travels down the length of the crystal and is detected by the photodiode. The photodiode converts the light into an electrical charge. This charge is stored until the thin-film transistor switches are electronically activated. When the switches are activated, the charged photodiode produces a signal that is read out and digitized.[3–8]

Like a flat-panel detector, a slot scanning detector uses a CsI (Tl) phosphor. In this type of detector, the CsI (Tl) phosphor is deposited on optical fibers that are connected to charge-coupled devices (CCDs). A CCD is an electronic chip that converts light photons to an electrical charge. As in a CsI flat-panel detector, x-rays strike the CsI (Tl) phosphor and are converted into light photons. The light photons pass down the crystal to the optical fibers. The light then travels through the optical fibers to the CCDs, which convert the light into an electronic signal that is digitized. The size of the CCDs limits the size of the detector. The CCDs in a slot scanning detector are placed together like tiles on a floor; the total area of the detector is thus relatively small compared with other types of detectors. The current commercially available slot scanning detector using this method is long and narrow. Because of this, the x-ray beam is collimated in a narrow slot

[*]President, Imorgan Medical, LLC, Menlo Park, California

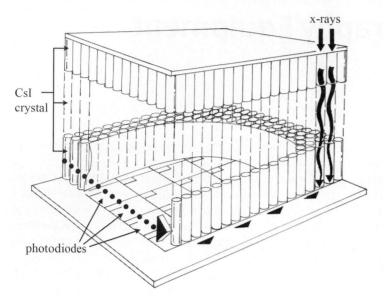

x-rays

CsI crystal

photodiodes

Figure 3–1 Schematic of a flat-panel cesium iodide (CsI) phosphor detector. The x-rays strike the CsI crystals and form light photons, which travel down the shaft of the crystal and strike a photodiode. The photodiode converts the light into an electrical charge. This charge is stored until the thin-film transistor switches (associated with each photodiode) are electronically activated. When the switches are activated, the charged photodiode produces a signal, which is read out and digitized.

to match the geometry of the detector. Also, because this type of detector is too narrow to read out information from the entire breast, the detector and the x-ray beam concurrently sweep across the breast. The image acquisition time in slot scanning detectors is longer than for other devices. This system requires a powerful x-ray tube and generator, as most of the x-rays are removed by the tight collimation. However, the collimation reduces scatter, and a grid is not necessary.

Selenium flat-panel detectors differ from CsI detectors in that the x-rays are directly converted into an electrical signal. This type of detector has three layers: an amorphous silicon base, an electrode pad central layer, and an amorphous selenium top layer. When x-rays hit the amorphous selenium, the selenium produces an electric charge by forming electron-hole pairs. An electric field is then applied between the electrodes, causing the electron-hole pairs to move to the polarized electrode. The charge created by these electron-hole pairs is read out on electrode pads that are laid on a plate of amorphous silicon. Because this system is not dependent on light photons, it is not subject to loss of resolution from divergence of light. Furthermore, the resolution of this method is not affected by the thickness of the photoconductor.

The third type of direct digital x-ray system is the quantum counting detector. This type counts each captured x-ray and converts them into signals. The process is fundamentally different from that employed in light phosphor detectors, which absorb x-rays and then produce an electric charge. The charge is proportional not only to the number of x-rays but also to the energy of the x-rays because more light is created by higher energy x-rays. If you wish to count all x-rays as equal, then you would need to count x-ray quanta. An example of a quantum counting detector is one that uses silicon crystals to receive x-rays. The charge is collected and then transformed into an electrical pulse. In another system, the captured x-rays convert a high-pressure gas to ions, and the ions form an electrical signal.[5]

CR mammographic acquisition systems are similar to those used for nonmammographic applications. X-rays that have passed through the breast temporarily free the electrons in the phosphor screen from the crystal matrix. These freed electrons are captured and stored in traps within the crystal lattice. The number of filled traps is proportional to the amount of absorbed x-rays. After the screen is exposed to x-rays, the technologist then places this phosphor screen in a reader. Within the reader, the screen is scanned by a red laser light, which liberates the electrons from the traps. The electrons then return to their original resting state (**Fig. 3–2**). As the electrons change state, they emit a blue light, which is measured by an optical collecting system that includes a photomultiplier tube. The blue light is proportional to the energy of x-rays absorbed by the phosphor. A filter prevents the red laser light from interfering with the measurement. The time the laser beam strikes a specific location corresponds to the x- and y-coordinates of each image location. The spatial sampling is determined by the laser spot size and the distance between sample measurements. The advantage of a CR system is that the phosphor plates are interchangeable with a conventional mammography unit, so the equipment cost may be lower than for other systems. Disadvantages include the need to transport the phosphor plates to a reader. Furthermore, scattering of red laser light during readout causes loss of resolution, as the light may cause adjacent phosphor areas to discharge.

Although digital mammographic systems differ according to the design of the detector, there are several features that all digital acquisition systems have in common. First of all, all acquisition systems have an operator's console that is used to control image acquisition. Also, acquisition systems usually have a viewing workstation that is used for quality control. This viewing workstation is different from the station used for image review.

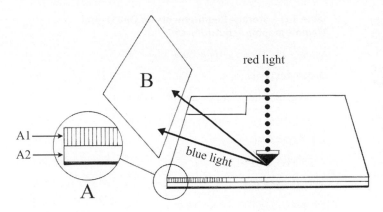

red light

B

A1 →
A2 →

blue light

A

Figure 3–2 Schematic of a computed radiology reader. X-rays passing through the breast free electrons in the phosphor screen. These electrons are then captured and stored in traps within the crystal lattice. The number of filled traps is proportional to the amount of absorbed x-rays. To read out the image, a technologist places the phosphor screen in a reader. Within the reader, the screen is scanned by a red laser light, which liberates the electrons from the traps and produces an emission of blue light, which is converted into an image.

In general, full-field digital systems have offered detector pixel resolution between 50 and 100 µ, field of views similar to screen-film (i.e., 24 × 30 cm), and also provide small spot image capability. Besides acquiring images, acquisition systems may do various types of image processing. Image processing usually includes setting window and level values. In addition, the system may superimpose proprietary processing that enhances image viewing.

Acquisition systems also package images in DICOM (Digital Imaging and Communications in Medicine) and send them to storage units and viewing stations. DICOM images sent from the acquisition system to storage use either the DICOM "Digital Mammography X-ray Image Storage—for presentation" or the "Digital Mammography X-ray Image Storage—for processing" class. These classes convey the same information, with the exception that the first conveys the intention that the image is for presentation, whereas the second conveys the intention that the image is for processing. Image acquisition systems with DICOM-conformant outputs can store images to any DICOM-conformant storage system that supports the digital mammographic DICOM classes.

■ Digital Image Display

Image display systems for diagnosis include one or more high-resolution monitors (usually two portrait orientation monitors), a computer, and image display software. The review station may use DICOM to retrieve images from the storage unit, or it may use a proprietary protocol. Image review stations typically provide the following functions:[11,12]

- *Study or patient list* This list allows the user to select a study for viewing. Sometimes the user may employ this list to select prior examinations for comparison. In some systems, this feature also allows the user to select studies performed in other modalities, such as ultrasound or magnetic resonance, and compare them to mammographic images.
- *Image placement protocols* This feature allows users to select a "hanging protocol." Generally, these protocols may be individualized. The protocols facilitate

rapid interpretation by automating the placement of images on the monitors.
- *Image display adjustment* Image display parameters may be changed. These adjustments include window and level settings. The window and level can usually be adjusted continuously or set to various preset values. Image magnification allows magnification of the entire image or a section of the image.
- *Postprocessing* Some workstations provide various postprocessing methods. These proprietary methods are intended to augment diagnosis by enhancing the visualization of the image.[9,10]
- *Computer-aided detection* Various types of computer-aided detection are being used to enhance the reading of mammography images. Not all workstations incorporate these functions.

In recent years, flat-panel displays have begun to replace cathode-ray tube (CRT) technology.[13] Today the best flat-panel displays can match or exceed the performance of CRT displays. Flat-panel display performance is expected to continue to improve, leading to the eventual obsolescence of CRT displays.

A typical FDA (Food and Drug Administration) 510(k) mammography–approved flat-panel display monitor has the following specifications:

- *Resolution* 2048 × 2560 (5 Mpixels)
- *Size* 21 inches diagonal
- *Pixel pitch* 165 µ
- *Brightness* 750 cd/m^2
- *Contrast ratio* 800:1
- *Palette* 3061 shades of gray (~12 bit gray scale). However, because the input is 8 bits, the monitor shows only 256 levels of gray.

The above information shows that the monitor will display a maximum of 5 Mpixels. Single-image sizes of CR, CsI, and selenium flat-plate detector systems range from 4 to 15 Mpixels.[4] Therefore, if the mammogram has more than 5 Mpixels, all the pixels within the image cannot be displayed at the same time. The number of pixels in the image must be reduced to display the entire image. This type of pixel reduction is known as image scaling. Scaling will reduce the image resolution. Alternatively, part of the image may be displayed at full resolution, allowing the user to pan to view all of the image. Currently, 5 Mpixel gray-scale monitors are the standard for mammography. However, as more acquisition units increase the number of pixels acquired per image, display requirements will probably become more demanding.[14] Higher pixel monitors are currently being clinically evaluated and will be available in the near future.

■ Digital Storage

Virtually all digital mammography acquisition systems will support DICOM storage and are able to store images in any DICOM system that supports the digital mammography DICOM requirements. Most DICOM storage systems are able to store digital mammography images because the digital mammography DICOM requirements are not significantly different from other types of DICOM storage classes.

However, because mammography images are unusually large, although a storage system can store a mammography image, it is not necessarily true that the storage system will work well in receiving and sending these large images quickly and efficiently.[15]

Assuming that a mammographic image is 24 × 30 cm, the pixel size is 100 μ, and the pixel depth is 16 bits, then a single image is ~14 MB in size. **Tables 3–1** and **3–2** give image size and storage requirements for images from a 100-μ (pixel spacing) sensor. This information assumes that the images are not compressed. If lossless compression is used, then storage requirements could be reduced by a factor of 2 to 3.

Image storage systems should be carefully designed to ensure that data are not lost and that continued operation is possible in the event of a storage system failure.

Picture Archiving and Communication System Technology and Mammography

Digital mammography can be completely freestanding and not integrated with other imaging systems. Initially, this organizational pattern was common because the modality

Table 3–1 Mammographic Image Size Requirements*

Sensor width	24 cm
Sensor length	30 cm
Sensor area	720 cm²
Pixel size	100 μ
Megapixels per image	7.2
Bits per pixel	16.0
Megabytes per image	14.4

*Requirements for images from a 100 μ sensor. Assumes images are not compressed.

Table 3–2 Storage Requirements for One Digital Mammographic Acquisition Unit

Assume: no. of images per study	5
Megabytes per study	72
Assume: no. of studies per hour per system	3
Studies per day	24
Studies per year	6000
Megabytes per year	432,000
Gigabytes per year	432
Storage cost dollars per gigabyte	$1.00
Cost to store 1 study	$0.07

was new and not supported by existing manufacturers of picture archiving and communication system (PACS) technology. Now that digital mammography is becoming more common, manufacturers are moving to incorporate support for digital mammography in their systems. This trend should continue because larger imaging organizations will prefer to incorporate digital mammography into their existing PACS units. Smaller imaging centers that do not have multimodality PACS may continue to use stand-alone systems. In hospitals and imaging centers that have PACS, there are strong reasons to incorporate digital mammography into the PACS setup:

- Reduced cost for storing mammography images by using an existing storage system
- Easier comparison of mammography images with images from other modalities
- Rapid distribution of images to various locations using existing PACS
- Reduced support costs of digital imaging
- Efficient sharing of workstations for different modalities

The transition from dedicated, stand-alone systems to multimodality PACS technology is facilitated by PACS vendors adding mammography review capabilities to their workstations. If you wish to integrate an existing PACS system with digital mammography, you will want to begin by reviewing the manufacturer's plans for digital mammographic integration. Compare the available PACS display features with digital mammographic features that are used daily. Because proprietary postprocessing from a digital mammographic system will not be available on a PACS system, you will need to learn if other comparable postprocessing techniques are available or if adequate window and level adjustments are attainable. Finally, you will need to evaluate the flexibility of the hanging protocols and identify sets that could be used for screening or diagnostic exams.

The main area of concern for incorporating digital mammography into a PACS infrastructure involves image processing. Currently, digital mammographic image processing is proprietary and may occur in the acquisition unit, the image display workstation, or the storage unit. In some systems, processing may occur at all of these locations. When purchasing a mammography system, it is very important to understand where this proprietary processing occurs in this particular system and what significance it has on the image. If this proprietary pattern is interrupted, clinical results may be suboptimal. This understanding is particularly important for imaging groups that may want to buy acquisition units from multiple vendors and have common workstations to interpret images from assorted units. This is also important for future migration to a new system. When an old digital system is replaced, even if the previous image was in a DICOM format, the radiologist may not be able to compare the previous exam successfully to images from the current equipment.[16,17]

In 2006, Integrating the Healthcare Enterprise (IHE), an initiative of health care professionals and industry to improve the way computer systems share information, developed standards for digital mammography.[18] IHE pro-motes the coordinated use of established standards such as DICOM and HL7 (Health Level 7) to allow seamless passage of information between medical providers. To facilitate workflow, the IHE profile dictates that mammographic images have encoded information that can be used by the workstation to determine hanging protocols; this allows current and prior exams to be automatically displayed. The actual organization of these protocols is not defined or determined, only the digital tools that may be used. Other examples of IHE standards are the requirements that workstations orient mammographic images according to laterality and are capable of justifying images to the chest-wall side so that mammograms may be viewed back-to-back.[19] Because the development of the IHE mammographic profile is relatively recent, there will be a transition period to allow manufacturers to conform to the new standards. Prospective buyers should inquire about a particular system's compliance with the IHE profile. For further information, consult the IHE Web site (http://www.ihe.net/index.cfm).

References

1. Ikeda DM. Mammographic acquisition: screen-film and digital mammography, computer-aided detection, and the mammography quality standards act. In: Breast Imaging: The Requisites. Philadelphia: Elsevier Mosby; 2004:1–23
2. Obenauer S, Luftner-Nagel S, Von Heyden D, Munzel U, Baum F, Grabbe E. Screen film vs. full-field digital mammography: image quality, detectability and characterization of lesions. Eur Radiol 2002;12:1697–1702
3. Pisano ED, Yaffe MJ. Digital mammography. Radiology 2005; 234:353–362
4. Mahesh M. AAPM/RSNA Physics tutorial for residents: digital mammography: an overview. Radiographics 2004;24:1747–1760
5. Yaffe MJ, Mainprize JG. Detectors for digital mammography. In: Pisano ED, Yaffe MJ, Kuzmiak CM, eds. Digital Mammography. Philadelphia: Lippincott Williams & Wilkins; 2003:15–32
6. D'Orsi CJ. Digital mammography: principles, equipment, technique, and clinical results. In: Feig SA, ed. Breast Imaging. Oak Brook, IL: RSNA; 2005:77–82
7. D'Orsi CJ. Digital mammography in the clinical practice. In: Karellas A, Giger ML, eds. Advances in Breast Imaging: Physics, Technology, and Clinical Applications. Oak Brook, IL: RSNA; 2004:87–100
8. Karellas A, Vedantham S, Suryanarayanan S. Digital mammography image acquisition technology. In: Karellas A, Giger ML, eds. Advances in Breast Imaging: Physics, Technology, and Clinical Applications. Oak Brook, IL: RSNA; 2004:87–100
9. Pisano ED, Cole EB, Major S, et al. Radiologists' preferences for digital mammographic display. Radiology 2000;216:820–830
10. Cole EB, Pisano ED, Kistner EO, et al. Diagnostic accuracy of digital mammography in patients with dense breasts who underwent problem-solving mammography: effects of image processing and lesion type. Radiology 2003;226:153–160
11. Hemminger BM. Soft copy display requirements for digital mammography. J Digit Imaging 2003;16:292–305
12. Suryanarayanan S, Karellas A, Vedantham S, Ved H, Baker SP, D'Orsi CJ. Flat-panel digital mammography system: contrast-detail comparison between screen-film radiographs and hard-copy images. Radiology 2002;225:801–807
13. Obenauer S, Hermann K-P, Marten K, et al. Soft copy versus hard copy reading in digital mammography. J Digit Imaging 2003;16:341–344
14. Samei E. Digital mammographic displays. In: Karellas A, Giger ML, eds. Advances in Breast Imaging: Physics, Technology, and Clinical Applications. Oak Brook, IL: RSNA; 2004:87–100
15. Jong RA, Yaffe MJ. Digital mammography: 2005. Can Assoc Radiol J 2005;56:319–323
16. Behlen FM. PACS issues. In: Pisano ED, Yaffe MJ, Kuzmiak CM, eds. Digital Mammography. Philadelphia: Lippincott Williams & Wilkins; 2003:62–66
17. Van Ongeval C, Bosmans H, Van Steen A. Current challenges of full field digital mammography. Radiat Prot Dosimetry 2005;117:148–153
18. ACC/HIMSS/RSNA. IHE radiology technical framework supplement, 2006–2007. Mammography image (MAMMO) integration profile. Available at: http://www. Ihe.net/technical_framework/upload/ IHE_RAD-RF_Suppl_MAMMO_TI_2006-04-13
19. Oosterwijk H, Cunie D. Digital mammography: the next frontier for IHE. Health Imaging and IT, June, 2006. Available at http://www. healthimaging.com/content/view/4390/84/

4 Normal Anatomy

■ Digital Mammographic Technique of Normal Breast

Normal breast anatomy is well displayed with digital mammography. The breast fibroglandular tissue is framed by numerous short arched lines. The internal pattern of the breast consists of fibroglandular tissue that forms a matrix of short curvilinear lines and longer trabecular lines that are oriented to the nipple. These lines coalesce to form a thin attachment to the nipple.

The skin and the subcutaneous tissues generally are more visible with digital mammography than with screen-film technique.[1,2] The skin is usually uniform and gradually thickens closer to the nipple. Variations in normal structures that are displayed by digital mammography can be confusing to imagers accustomed to screen-film displays. Although the nipple-areolar complex is generally symmetric bilaterally, there is sometimes normal or chronic asymmetric skin thickening or nipple inversion. Asymmetry may be due to poor patient positioning or compression. Even with good technique, the nipple-areolar complex may be asymmetric. In these cases, it is important to evaluate closely the skin, nipple,

and subareolar fibroglandular tissue. On screening digital images, you can magnify, window, and level the display of this area to search for asymmetries, suspicious calcifications, or architectural distortion. Old films, even if they are screen-film, are useful for comparison because the asymmetry may prove to be chronic. If the patient is recalled, the nipple and skin should be visually inspected and compared with the contralateral side, and the patient should be questioned concerning nipple irritation, discharge, or skin changes. Spot magnification views are more sensitive for identifying subtle architectural distortions or suspicious calcifications. Besides providing better display of the skin and nipple, digital mammography is better at revealing structures in the retromammary space. Furthermore, digital mammography produces better image contrast and exposure with fewer artifacts.[1,2] However, like screen-film mammography, digital mammography still requires monitoring for adequate clinical quality (**Fig. 4–1**).

Every year, the number of postprocessing methods and hanging protocol options available on digital workstations grows. The numerous choices may be daunting to those who are faced with developing a display protocol for the first time. One way to develop a protocol is to observe

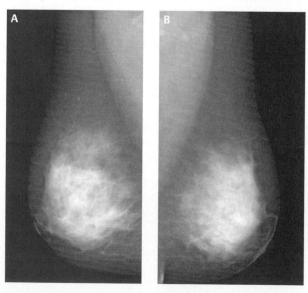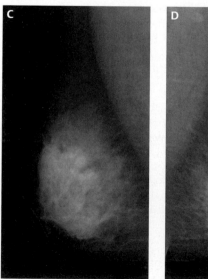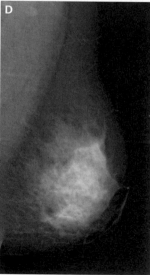

Figure 4–1 Mediolateral oblique (MLO) views. **(A)** Right MLO, **(B)** left MLO with grid lines, **(C)** right MLO, and **(D)** left MLO without grid lines. This study had been started when the technologist immediately noted that there were grid lines in the image that were due to improper lack of movement of the grid. After the grid mechanism was fixed, the lines were no longer present.

the activities that are currently performed when reading mammograms. These activities will vary depending on whether screening or diagnostic mammograms are being read. Additionally, the frequency of activities should be noted. For example, an activity that is performed on 100% of screening mammograms should clearly be part of a routine protocol. An activity that is performed less than 10% of the time may be omitted from the protocol and performed as needed.

Initially, a screening protocol includes display of the four screening views. For soft copy digital screening, a preferred postprocessing program should be identified as the default for all screening exams to avoid missing any subtle abnormalities. The radiologist should then review these images in the same manner that the imager scans screen-film images.

The current screening views are then displayed with a previous screening exam. If earlier exams are recorded on film, the radiologist reads the film from a multiviewer or light box adjacent to the soft copy workstation. The monitors should be adjusted to minimize reflected glare. If earlier exams are digital, then the earlier exam should be compared side by side on the digital soft copy display monitors.

There are several different methods that can be used to display current and old exams. If you prefer large images, then the two mediolateral oblique (MLO) views from the earlier exam can be placed next to the two current exam MLOs on two monitors. If you do not mind smaller images, you may prefer to see four views—two craniocaudal (CC) views and two MLOs—from the earlier exam compared with the four views (two CCs and two MLOs) in the current exam; these eight images may be displayed in two horizontal rows, each containing four images. The actual size of each image is only slightly smaller than the usual screen-film image. When comparing the current exam to earlier exams, you can identify any subtle new asymmetry and assess the chronicity of lesions that have been identified with the initial evaluation of the screening views.

Finally, magnification of the current exam should be incorporated into the viewing protocol. Magnification can be performed in several ways, depending on the display workstation being used. These choices include manually magnifying a small region or automated enlargement of large sections of the breast. Prior to magnification, you can apply a proprietary postprocessing technique, choose a higher full-resolution mode, or reverse the black/white gray scale. Choose the method in which you can efficiently perform a comprehensive examination of the whole breast. Obviously, magnification may be performed at any time during the examination. By routinely performing this action last, you can cluster the evaluation of all potentially suspicious lesions and save time. If asymmetries or masses are present, you

can adjust the brightness and contrast to characterize them. Although digital display workstations provide a variety of display techniques, if a potentially suspicious mammographic abnormality is present on the screening exam, the patient should be recalled for additional mammographic examination.[3]

Imaging protocols for diagnostic mammography are more complex than screening exams. Depending on the flexibility of the digital workstation capabilities, the systematic display of diagnostic images may be problematic. In general, for a dual-monitor digital workstation, if the diagnostic examination consists of fewer than five spot compression or magnification images, then the simplest method is to display these images on one monitor and display the original two or four screening images on the second monitor. If the diagnostic exam, including pertinent original screening images, consists of fewer than nine "full-size" images (e.g., rolled views, 90-degree lateral view, and shallow obliques), then the images may be displayed in one or two horizontal rows. In each of these scenarios, if you do not wish to examine four images on one monitor, you may either evaluate the additional images separately from the original screening images or analyze each side separately, depending on the clinical situation.

■ General Mammographic Evaluation

The mammographic report for digital mammography has the same five elements as that of screen-film: (1) indication for the exam; (2) description of breast composition; (3) explanation of significant findings; (4) comparison with previous exams; and (5) general impression, which incorporates a Breast Imaging Reporting and Data System (BI-RADS) assessment category.[4] Examples of indications for examinations include screening, identification of a clinical finding, such as a palpable lump, and following a patient who has been treated for breast cancer.

Breast composition is quantitatively described by the BI-RADS. The categories of composition are (1) almost entirely fat, (2) scattered fibroglandular densities, (3) heterogeneously dense, and (4) extremely dense.[4] Breast tissue that is almost entirely fat consists of less than 25% fibroglandular tissue. Although this type of tissue is easiest to identify suspicious lesions, it is important that the display has adequate image contrast. With a fatty background, poor contrast may be overlooked because skin and trabecular lines appear to be relatively bright (**Figs. 4–2**).

When scattered fibroglandular densities are present, the breast tissue is composed of 25 to 50% glandular tissue (**Figs. 4–3** and **4–4**). Mammograms exhibiting

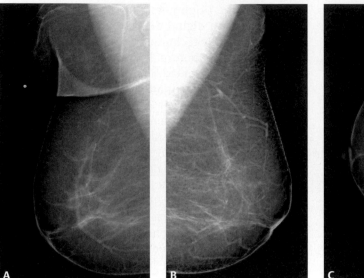

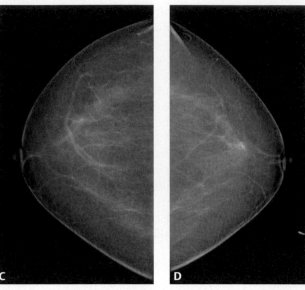

Figure 4–2 Mediolateral oblique (MLO) and craniocaudal (CC) views. **(A)** Right MLO, **(B)** left MLO, **(C)** right CC, and **(D)** left CC mammograms. In this case, the patient presented with soft palpable fullness in the right axilla. Mammograms demonstrate that the breasts are composed almost entirely of fat. Mammographically, the patient has asymmetric fatty tissue in the right axilla. Differential includes accessory breast tissue or asymmetric fat. (Sonographic exam demonstrated only fat. Physical exam was benign.) Left axilla is normal.

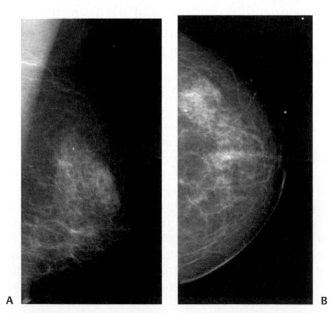

Figure 4–3 Mediolateral oblique (MLO) and craniocaudal (CC) views. **(A)** Left MLO and **(B)** CC mammograms. Left screening mammograms demonstrate the breast is composed of benign scattered fibroglandular densities.

fibroglandular volumes in the lower half of this range are easier to recognize compared with the upper half (i.e., 40–50% fibroglandular volume) of this category. A method to separate this from the next composition category (i.e., heterogeneously dense breast) is related to the amount of tissue that one can "see through." Subjectively, a breast with 40 to 50% fibroglandular volume is filled with a mixture of fatty and glandular tissue. However, very little of this fibroglandular volume represents completely opacified breast tissue (i.e., tissue that would completely obscure any mass).

Breasts that are heterogeneously dense have ~51 to 75% of the breast obscured by breast tissue, and extremely dense breasts consist of more than 75% glandular tissue. Mammograms with both heterogeneously dense or extremely dense composition suggest that lesions may be obscured by the surrounding fibroglandular density in these mammograms (**Figs. 4–5**). Studies have shown that digital mammography reduces fibroglandular opacity; therefore, mammographic composition of patients with heterogeneous or extremely dense breasts appears less dense on digital mammography compared with screen-film mammography. Researchers have found that this reduction in density leads to greater confidence in excluding masses in these dense breasts. However, the digital mammographic detection rate of cancers (and masses) in these studies is equivalent to screen-film technique.[2,5]

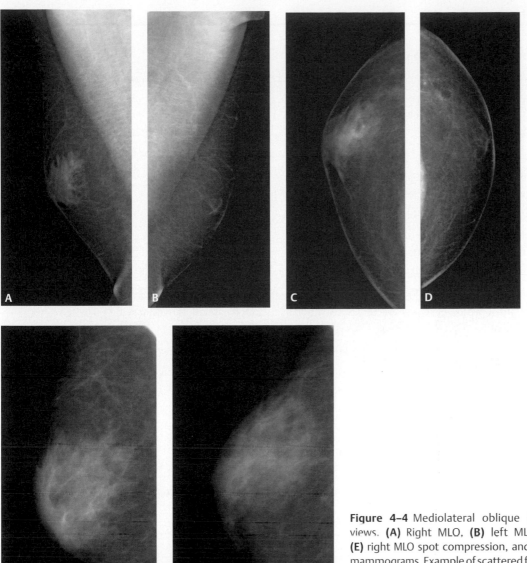

Figure 4–4 Mediolateral oblique (MLO) and craniocaudal (CC) views. **(A)** Right MLO, **(B)** left MLO, **(C)** right CC, **(D)** left CC, **(E)** right MLO spot compression, and **(F)** right CC spot compression mammograms. Example of scattered fibroglandular composition in the right breast and fatty composition in the left breast of a male patient. Like female fibroglandular tissue, male tissue is composed of curvilinear densities infiltrated with oval fatty lucencies. The central subareolar tissue on the right is consistent with benign gynecomastia.

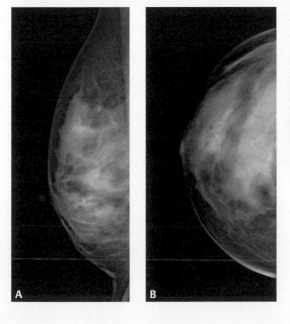

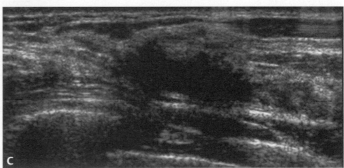

Figure 4–5 Mediolateral (MLO and craniocaudal (CC) views. **(A)** Right MLO and **(B)** right CC mammograms. In this case, the patient presented with a palpable right breast mass. She had mammographically heterogeneously dense breast composition, so it was not surprising that the palpable lump that is evident on a sonogram **(C)** is mammographically occult.

Table 4–1 Summary BI-RADS Assessments for Mammography

BI-RADS Assessment	Definition	Likelihood of Malignancy
Category 0	Need additional imaging evaluation and/or prior mammograms for comparison	
Category 1	Negative	
Category 2	Benign finding	
Category 3	Probably benign finding; initial short-term interval follow-up suggested	Less than 2%
Category 4	Suspicious abnormality—biopsy should be considered	
Category 4A (optional)	Malignant pathology not expected: 6-month or routine follow-up after benign biopsy	Low suspicion: ~3 to 33%
Category 4B (optional)	Follow-up benign biopsy result depends on pathologic/radiologic concordance	Intermediate risk of malignancy about 34 to 64%
Category 4C (optional)	Malignant pathology result expected; close pathologic evaluation of benign pathologic results	Moderate risk of malignancy: ~65 to 94%
Category 5	Highly suspicious of malignancy—appropriate action recommended	High risk of malignancy $\geq$ 95%
Category 6	Known biopsy proven malignancy—appropriate action recommended	Biopsy proven malignancy

BI-RADS, Breast Imaging Reporting and Data System.

Source: Breast imaging and reporting data system—mammography. In: D'Orsi CJ, Bassett LW, Berg WA, et al, eds. BI-RADS Breast Imaging Reporting and Data System. Preston, VA: American College of Radiology; 2003:1–336. Reprinted with permission.

After evaluation of each digital mammographic examination, the radiologist summarizes the digital examination with the same BI-RADS assessment categories as screen-film (**Table 4–1**).

References

1. Obenauer S, Luftner-Nagel S, Heyden DV, Munzel U, Baum F, Grabbe E. Screen film vs. full-field mammography: image quality, detectability and characterization of lesions. Eur Radiol 2002;12:1697–1702
2. Fischmann A, Siegmann KC, Wersebe A, Claussen CD, Muller-Schimplfle M. Comparison of full-field digital mammography and film-screen mammography: image quality and lesion detection. Br J Radiol 2005;78:312–315
3. Fischer U, Hermann KP, Baum F. Digital mammography: current state and future aspects. Eur Radiol 2006;16:38–44
4. Breast imaging and reporting data system—mammography. In: D'Orsi CJ, Bassett LW, Berg WA, et al, eds. BI-RADS Breast Imaging Reporting and Data System. Preston, VA: American College of Radiology; 2003:1–336
5. Venta LA, Hendrick RE, Adler YT, . Rates and causes of disagreement in interpretation of full-field digital mammography and film-screen mammography in a diagnostic setting. AJR Am J Roentgenol 2001;176:1241–1248

5 Digital Mammographic Appearance of Benign and Malignant Calcifications

■ Digital Mammographic Technique for Calcifications

Detecting breast microcalcifications is one of the most important ways to identify breast cancer. Fifty to 80% of breast cancers have microscopic calcifications.[1] Furthermore, clustered microcalcifications consist of up to 40% of non-palpable cancers.[2] Because the spatial resolution of digital mammography is poorer than screen-film mammography, there has been concern that digital mammography is less sensitive in displaying malignant microcalcifications compared with screen-film. Whereas the spatial resolution of screen-film mammography is greater than 15 line pairs per mm (lp/mm), digital mammography units have been found to have a spatial resolution as low as 5 lp/mm. Despite the reduced spatial resolution, studies have reported that digital mammographic units display simulated microcalcifications within phantoms in a manner that is at least comparable to screen-film machines.[3] This relative equivalence in diagnostic detectability applies to the comparison of digital spot mammography with conventional spot mammography.[4] Researchers from the M. D. Anderson Cancer Center (Houston, Texas) have found that within a breast phantom that has a uniform background, digital flat-panel mammographic units perform better than conventional screen-film mammography units in identifying particles that simulate microcalcifications.[5] After magnification is added to the imaging devices, the performance of conventional screen-film equipment becomes equivalent to digital flat-panel mammography. When the simulated calcifications are placed within a phantom with a background that simulates complex breast tissue, the screen-film and the digital charge-coupled device unit initially perform better. However, magnification substantially improves the performance of the digital flat-panel mammographic unit, so that there is no significant difference. Although microcalcifications may be visible with larger pixel digital images, Ruschin et al noted that increasing pixel size is associated with decreasing the ability of radiologists to identify the shape of the microcalcifications.[6]

Multiple retrospective studies have been performed to compare the visibility of microcalcifications using digital mammography with conventional screen-film mammography. Fischer and colleagues compared the appearance of 37 cases of microcalcifications (21 malignant, 16 benign) that had been documented with screen-film mammography and digital mammography hard copy filmed images.[7]

They reported that all breast imagers had a slightly higher sensitivity and specificity for the calcifications using the digital mammographic images compared with the screen-film images, but this difference was not statistically significant. Multiple clinical investigators using soft copy review of digital images have reinforced these findings: receiver operator characteristic analysis indicates that the performance of breast imagers using digital mammography is better compared with screen-film. However, these differences are not statistically significant.[8–10] As radiologists become more experienced and as the equipment advances, digital mammographic evaluation of calcifications will continue to improve. Kim et al reported that after comparing the image quality, number, and conspicuity of 40 clustered calcifications (3 malignant, 37 benign), radiologists judged soft copy digital mammographic images as better in all categories compared with screen-film exams.[11]

When using digital mammography, a routine method to evaluate the breast for microcalcifications should be incorporated into screening. If hard copy film is being used to review digital mammograms, the routine will probably be similar to the screen-film mammographic method. However, if a soft copy display is being used, then a digital imaging method is preferable. The initial identification may involve a rapid review of the four screening views using a presentation size that is at least equivalent to that used in mammographic film. Because of the flexibility of soft copy display, the screening views can be displayed at a size larger than film. Once the screening views are reviewed, the display can be magnified to specifically identify calcifications. This manipulation would be comparable to using a magnification glass with screen-film. Before enlarging or magnifying the image, the radiologist may prefer to superimpose a proprietary higher contrast display mode or a high-resolution mode. Magnification may be performed by sweeping the image with a small field of view (FOV) digital magnifying glass or by magnifying large segments of the image (e.g., a quadrant or a third of the image).

Computer-aided detection (CAD) is commonly used in conjunction with digital mammographic screening exams. Although each CAD system uses different labels, all manufacturers have annotations that denote the presence of possible microcalcifications. Multiple studies have shown that CAD programs tend to perform better in identifying malignant microcalcifications compared with masses.[12,13]

Retrospective studies have suggested that CAD has an excellent receiver operating characteristics curve and that it may reduce interoperator variability.[14-16] More experienced readers probably benefit less from CAD than do less experienced interpreters.[17] However, even with the use of CAD, the radiologist still bears the primary responsibility for identifying suspicious calcifications, as CAD is not sensitive in identifying less conspicuous depositions, such as amorphous calcifications.[18]

CAD results can be viewed either at the beginning or at the end of the screening examination. By viewing the CAD images early, the radiologist can incorporate the examination of any suspected CAD calcifications into a routine screening evaluation. If CAD images are viewed at the end of the screening examination, the radiologist should plan to reevaluate the breast for CAD-identified calcifications that were initially missed. With experience, the radiologist will miss few CAD-identified significant microcalcifications.

Once calcifications are identified, digital mammography offers an array of new methods to examine microcalcifications. In general, when examining calcifications, the highest resolution available on a particular system should be used. Furthermore, a display mode should be used that allows the operator to characterize the shape of the calcifications. Alternatively, the window and gray scale can be manipulated manually. If the cluster is extremely small, multiple magnification levels should be performed until the morphology of the calcifications is discernible. If the calcifications are distributed regionally or segmentally, it may be best to magnify a larger portion of the breast, such as a quadrant, with an automated format. Some imagers prefer to invert the white/black/gray scale when examining calcifications. One of the strengths of digital mammography is the ability of the imager to match the display of the current image to the appearance of earlier digital examinations to assess the stability of calcifications. Although there may be slight differences in compression and patient position, generally the imager can rapidly localize the area on a previous image and match the contrast and magnification. This flexibility is particularly useful for evaluating clustered punctate calcifications.

Although many digital techniques can be applied to the examination of calcifications, it is still useful to recall the patient to perform additional magnification views. Orthogonal views, such as mediolateral views, are useful to confirm the location of subtle calcifications. Mammographic images that examine the periphery of the breast, such as exaggerated craniocaudal views, are useful when the calcifications are visible on only one view. Magnification digital views have superior spatial resolution to screening digital images and generally demonstrate the calcification shapes more clearly than the screening examination. Finally, even with highly suspicious calcifications, magnification views are useful to map the extent of disease. This information is important when discussing pretreatment chemotherapy options or planning needle localization bracketing prior to excision.

General Evaluation of Mammographic Calcifications

When faced with assessing calcifications, it is important to have a clear clinical strategy that should be similar to the one used for screen-film mammography. In general, most clinical strategies involve assessing specific characteristics of the calcifications, including size, distribution, and shape. The author's personal approach is to decide first if the calcifications are benign. This approach to evaluating calcifications rests upon answering three key questions: (1) Are the calcifications large? (2) Is the distribution of calcifications diffuse or scattered? and (3) Do they belong to a special group of calcifications that are synonymous with benignity? If the answer to any of these three questions is yes, then the calcifications are benign, as defined by category 2 of the Breast Imaging Reporting and Data System (BI-RADS). If a set of calcifications is determined to be benign, then the workup is finished. Inexperienced radiology residents will commonly forget this rule and start to work up benign calcifications.

Benign calcifications are generally larger than 0.5 mm. If the calcification is larger than 2 mm, then it is almost certainly benign. In general, because benign calcifications are larger than malignant calcifications, they are relatively readily identified on digital mammography without magnification.

Scattered or diffuse distribution is also usually associated with benign calcifications. The exception is when the patient has extensive involvement with ductal carcinoma in situ (DCIS) or a combination of invasive ductal and DCIS. However, usually this would not be confused with benign disease because, in this situation, the morphology of the calcifications is compatible with a highly suspicious lesion.

There are several types of benign calcifications with a well-established morphology. These include vascular calcifications, milk of calcium, skin calcifications, lucent center calcifications, secretory calcifications, and popcorn calcifications of fibroadenomas. Eggshell and rim calcifications are grouped within the classification of lucent center calcifications. Although each of these types has a classic presentation, when they are early in development, they may not have a pathognomonic appearance and may appear suspicious.

If calcifications are determined to be smaller than 0.5 mm, not scattered, and do not have a distinctively benign morphology, they must be inspected closely. The most common types of calcifications in this category are punctate, amorphous, coarse heterogeneous, fine pleomorphic, fine linear, and fine linear branching. Of these, the least suspicious are the punctate calcifications. Clustered punctate are the most common calcifications defined as probably benign (category 3) using BI-RADS. This category contains lesions with a low (<2%) chance of malignancy. Such microcalcifications may be observed with close-interval mammographic follow-up examinations. In the fourth edition of BI-RADS,[19] punctate calcifications are differentiated from round calcifications by their size. Punctate calcifications are smaller than 0.5 mm, and round calcifications are larger than 0.5 mm. Generally, round calcifications less than 1 mm in diameter are within the acini of lobules and are considered benign. However, if they are new and clustered, they warrant being closely followed. New clustered punctate calcifications should also be assessed as category 3. The reason for the close follow-up is that DCIS may occasionally present with round or punctate calcifications. Therefore, if these calcifications increase in number or transform into a suspicious morphology, they should be assessed as BI-RADS category 4 (suspicious), and biopsy is justified. If the calcifications are stable for 2 years, they may be assessed as BI-RADS category 2 (benign), and the patient may return to routine mammographic screening.

If a cluster of any of the other described morphologies (i.e., amorphous, coarse heterogeneous, fine pleomorphic, fine linear, or fine linear branching) is identified, these calcifications should be assessed as either BI-RADS category 4 (suspicious; biopsy should be considered) or category 5 (highly suggestive of malignancy; appropriate action should be taken). Although, in general, all of these suspicious calcifications are referred for biopsy prior to definitive therapy, accurate assessment is important for histologic radiologic correlation after biopsy. In higher risk lesions, if the preliminary microscopic diagnosis is benign, the radiologist will be more aggressive in determining if the lesion has been adequately sampled and microscopically examined.

Because of the importance of cross-correlation between histology and mammographic findings, risk assessment is part of the BI-RADS assessment system. Until the fourth edition of BI-RADS, it was more difficult to correlate the category 4 assessment to biopsy results. This was because the category 4 assessment previously included a wide probability of risk. Because category 3 represents lesions that have a less than 2% risk of malignancy[19] and the category 5 abnormalities have an extremely high (≥95% probability)[19] chance of malignancy, the category 4 assessment included probabilities between 3 and 94%. To clarify assessment, the BI-RADS now divides category 4 into three subcategories: category 4A (low suspicion: 3–33%), category 4B (intermediate suspicion: ~34–64%), and category 4C (moderate suspicion: ~65–94%). **Table 5–1** summarizes the various BI-RADs categories.[18,20,21]

There is considerable overlap risk when the calcifications are stratified by shape alone. In general, fine linear or fine linear branching are associated with the highest risk of malignancy.[22-24] However, besides calcification shape, distribution of calcifications will alter the assessment. In particular, linear or segmental distribution increases the probability of malignancy of moderately suspicious calcifications.[20,25] For example, although the most common category 5 lesion is the fine linear or branching calcifications, sometimes a patient presents with a segmental or linear distribution of fine pleomorphic calcifications, which warrants a category 5 assessment.

Although BI-RADS establishes a definition of calcification shape, the clinical description of calcifications is subject to inter- and intraobserver variance.[26,27] Researchers are devising methods to objectify the BI-RADS descriptions that will improve the positive predictive value of biopsy rates and better identify histologic results that are discordant with mammographic findings.[28,29]

Table 5–1   Summary of BI-RADS Assessments for Mammographic Calcifications

BI-RADS Assessment	Definition	Examples of Mammographic Calcification Findings
Category 2	Benign finding	Large size (>0.5 mm) Scattered distribution Pathognomonic shape or appearance (e.g., vascular, milk of calcium, skin calcifications)
Category 3	Probably benign—initial short-term interval follow-up suggested	Clustered punctate calcifications
Category 4	Suspicious abnormality—biopsy should be considered	
Category 4A		Clustered punctate calcifications (increasing in number); clustered amorphous calcifications
Category 4B		Amorphous calcifications (segmental distribution or larger); coarse heterogeneous calcifications (clustered)
Category 4C		Fine pleomorphic calcifications (clustered)
Category 5	Highly suggestive of malignancy; appropriate action should be taken	Fine pleomorphic calcifications (linear or segmental distribution); fine linear, fine linear branching calcifications

BI-RADS, Breast Imaging Reporting and Data System.

References

1. Ikeda DM. Mammographic analysis of breast calcifications. In: Ikeda DM, ed. Breast Imaging: The Requisites. Philadelphia: Elsevier Mosby; 2004:60–89
2. Sickels EA. Mammographic features of 300 consecutive nonpalpable breast cancers. Am J Roentgenol 1986;146:661–663
3. Rong XJ, Shaw CC, Johnston DA, et al. Microcalcification detectability for four mammographic detectors: flat-panel, CCD, CR, and screen/film. Med Phys 2002;29:2052–2061
4. Yip WM, Pang SY, Yim WS, Kwok CS. ROC curve analysis of lesion detectability on phantoms: comparison of digital spot mammography with conventional spot mammography. Br J Radiol 2001;74: 621–628
5. Lai C-J, Shaw CC, Whitman GJ, et al. Visibility of simulated microcalcifications—a hardcopy-based comparison of three mammographic systems. Med Phys 2005;32:182–194
6. Ruschin M, Hemdal B, Andersson I, et al. Threshold pixel size for shape determination of microcalcifications in digital mammography: a pilot study. Radiat Prot Dosimetry 2005;114:415–423
7. Fischer U, Baum F, Obenauer S, et al. Comparative study in patients with microcalcifications: full-field digital mammography vs screen-film mammography. Eur Radiol 2002;12:2679–2683
8. Bonardi R, Ambrogetti D, Ciatto S, et al. Conventional versus digital mammography in the analysis of screen-detected lesions with low positive predictive value. Eur J Radiol 2005;55:258–263
9. Kim HH, Pisano ED, Cole EB, et al. Comparison of calcifications specificity in digital mammography using soft-copy display versus screen-film mammography. Am J Roentgenol 2006;187:47–50
10. Skaane P, Balleyguier C, Diekmann F, et al. Breast lesion detection and classification: comparison of screen-film mammography and full-field digital mammography with soft-copy reading—observer performance study. Radiology 2005;237:37–44
11. Kim HS, Han B-K, Choo K-S, Jeon YH, Kim J-H, Choe YH. Screen-film mammography and soft-copy full-field digital mammography: comparison in patients with microcalcifications. Korean J Radiol 2005;6:214–220
12. Warren Burhenne LJ, Wood SA, D'Orsi CJ, et al. Potential contribution of computer-aided detection to the sensitivity of screening mammography. Radiology 2003;215:554–562
13. Morton MJ, Whaley DH, Brandt KR, Amrami KK. Screening mammograms: interpretation with computer-aided detection—prospective evaluation. Radiology 2006;239:375–383
14. Kouskos E, Markopoulos C, Revenas I, et al. Computer-aided preoperative diagnosis of microcalcifications on mammograms. Acta Radiol 2003;44:43–46
15. Lauria A, Palmiero R, Forni G, et al. A study on two different CAD systems for mammography as an aid to radiological diagnosis in the search of microcalcification clusters. Eur J Radiol 2005;55:264–269
16. Jiang Y, Nishikawa RM, Schmidt RA, Toledano AY, Doi K. Potential of computer-aided diagnosis to reduce variability in radiologists' interpretations of mammograms depicting microcalcifications. Radiology 2001;220:787–794
17. Brem RF, Schoonjans JM. Radiologist detection of microcalcifications with and without computer-aided detection: a comparative study. Clin Radiol 2001;56:150–154
18. Soo MS, Rosen EL, Xia JQ, Ghate S, Baker JA. Computer-aided detection of amorphous calcifications. Am J Roentgenol 2005;184:887–892
19. Breast imaging reporting and data system—mammography. In: D'Orsi CJ, Bassett LW, Berg WA, Feig SA, Jackson VP, Kopans DB, et al, eds. BI-RADS Breast Imaging Reporting and Data System. Preston, VA: American College of Radiology; 2003:1–336
20. Liberman L, Abramson AF, Squires FB, Glassman JR, Morris EA, Dershaw DD. The breast imaging reporting and data system: positive predictive value of mammographic features and final assessment categories. Am J Roentgenol 1998;171:35–40
21. Berg WA, Arnoldus CL, Teferra E, Bhargavan M. Biopsy of amorphous breast calcifications: pathologic outcome and yield at stereotactic biopsy. Radiology 2001;221:495–503
22. Alberdi E, Taylor P, Lee R, Rox J, Todd-Pokkropek A. Eliciting a terminology for mammographic calcifications. Clin Radiol 2002;57:1007–1013
23. Stomper PC, Connolly JL. Ductal carcinoma in situ of the breast: correlation between mammographic calcification and tumor subtype. Am J Roentgenol 1992;159:483–485
24. Gulsun M, Basaran DF, Ariyurek M. Evaluation of breast microcalcifications according to Breast Imaging Reporting and Data System criteria and Le Gal's classification. Eur J Radiol 2003;47:227–231
25. Barreau B, de Mascarel I, Feuga C, et al. Mammography of ductal carcinoma in situ of the breast: review of 909 cases with radiographic-pathologic correlations. Eur J Radiol 2005;54:55–61
26. Berg WA, Campassi C, Langenberg P, Sexton MJ. Breast Imaging Reporting and Data System: inter- and intraobserver variability in feature analysis and final assessment. Am J Roentgenol 2000;174:1769–1777
27. Lazarus E, Mainiero MB, Schepps B, Koeliker SL, Livingston LS. BI-RADS lexicon for US and mammography: interobserver variability and positive predictive value. Radiology 2006;239:385–391
28. Burnside ES, Rubin DL, Shachter RD, Sohlich RE, Sickles EA. A probabilistic expert system that provides automated mammographic-histologic correlation: initial experience. Am J Roentgenol 2004;182:481–488
29. Burnside ES, Rubin DL, Fine JP, Shachter RD, Sisney GA, Leung WK. Bayesian network to predict breast cancer risk of mammographic microcalcifications and reduce number of benign biopsy results: initial experience. Radiology 2006;240:666–673
30. Lagios MD. Multicentricity of breast carcinoma demonstrated by routine correlated serial subgross and radiographic examination. Cancer 1977;40:1726–1734

■ Case 5–1

Calcification Morphology   Skin calcifications

Distribution of Calcifications   Diffuse/scattered

Clinical History   A 64-year-old woman who has had bilateral breast cancers presents for screening.

Physical Examination   Normal exam

Radiologic Findings

Mammography

Figure 5–1 Mediolateral (ML) and craniocaudal (CC) views. **(A)** Left ML magnified tangential and **(B)** left CC magnified tangential mammograms. There are scattered punctate and round calcifications in the inferior breast. These magnified tangential views demonstrate that the calcifications are within the skin.

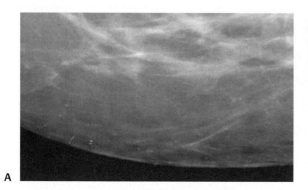
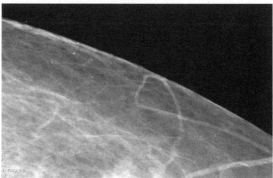

A   B

Management   BI-RADS category 2, benign finding

Pathologic Diagnosis

Benign

Skin calcifications

Pearls and Pitfalls

- Digital mammography is particularly better than screen-film mammography in identifying skin calcifications. If it is unclear whether the calcifications are within the skin, an electronic grid can be used to localize the calcifications while the patient is still in compression; a radiopaque marker is then placed on the skin over the position of the calcifications. Using this marker, a tangential magnified image of the skin is taken. Because digital mammography does not require film processing, it is much faster than screen-film mammography.

■ Case 5–2

Calcification Morphology   Skin calcifications

Distribution of Calcifications   Diffuse/scattered

Clinical History   A 56-year-old woman presents for screening.

Physical Examination   Normal exam

Radiologic Findings

Mammography

Figure 5–2 Mediolateral oblique (MLO) and craniocaudal (CC) views. **(A)** Right MLO, **(B)** right CC, **(C)** right CC magnification, **(D)** right MLO magnification, and **(E)** right MLO magnification with white and black inverted. At the 3 o'clock position in the right breast, there are some scattered round and oval calcifications with lucent centers. The magnification CC view **(C)** demonstrates that the calcifications are within the skin.

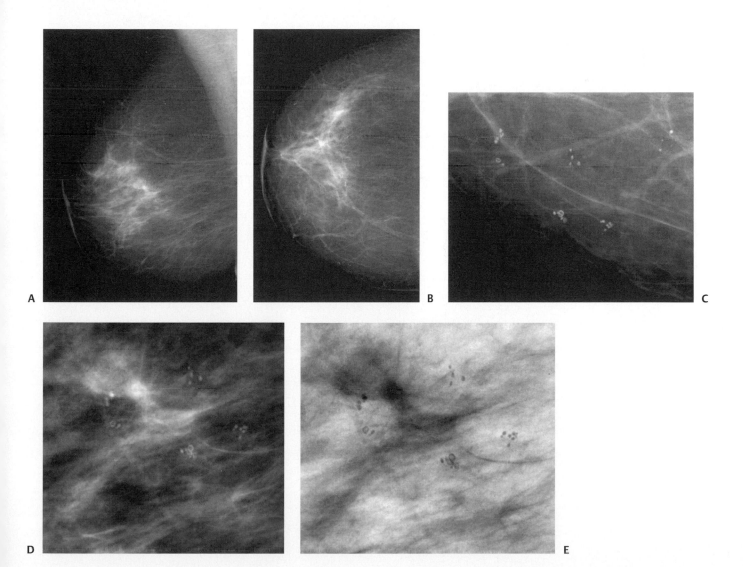

Management   BI-RADS category 2, benign finding

Pathologic Diagnosis

Benign

Skin calcifications

Pearls and Pitfalls

- Besides highly magnifying images, digital mammography can invert the black-and-white presentation, which sometimes clarifies the appearance of calcifications. In this case, the skin calcifications exhibit pathognomonic lucent centers.

■ Case 5–3

Calcification Morphology   Skin calcifications

Clinical History   A 59-year-old woman presents for screening.

Physical Examination   Normal exam

Radiologic Findings

Mammography

Figure 5–3 Mediolateral oblique (MLO) and craniocaudal (CC) views. **(A)** Right MLO, **(B)** right CC, and **(C)** right MLO digitally enlarged. In the right inferior outer breast, there are scattered punctate calcifications. With digital magnification of the screening views **(C)**, it can be seen that these calcifications are within the skin.

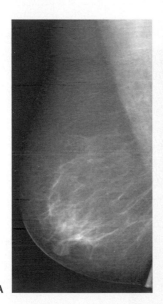
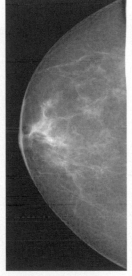
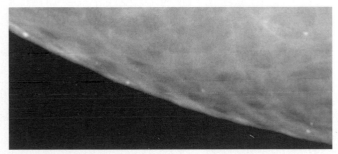

A   B   C

Management   BI-RADS category 2, benign finding

Pathologic Diagnosis

Benign

Skin calcifications

Pearls and Pitfalls

- This case illustrates that digital mammography increases the flexibility of the radiologist to analyze screening mammograms. The skin calcifications could be easily identified on the screening views. Usually, skin calcifications are not identified with screen-film technique because the skin is too dark.
- The MLO used for illustrating this case did not demonstrate the nipple in profile. An additional MLO had been performed with acceptable positioning, but this MLO demonstrated the benign calcifications better.

■ Case 5–4

Calcification Morphology   Miscellaneous

Clinical History   A 44-year-old woman presents for screening.

Physical Examination   Normal exam

Radiologic Findings

Mammography

Figure 5–4 Mediolateral oblique (MLO) views. **(A)** Left MLO mammogram and **(B)** enlargement of axillary section of MLO mammogram. There is a thick, coarse linear density in the axilla that is visible only on the MLO view. **(C)** Left MLO mammogram. After cleaning the axilla, the linear density has disappeared, consistent with skin contamination, such as deodorant.

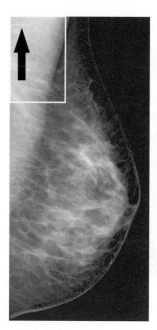 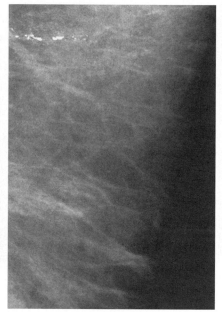 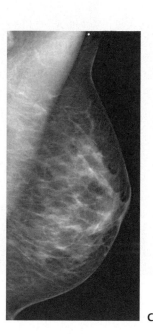

A   B   C

Management   BI-RADS category 2, benign finding

Pathologic Diagnosis

Benign

Deodorant

Pearls and Pitfalls

- Antiperspirants commonly contain aluminum, which may produce mammographic densities. Other skin creams containing metallic compounds, such as zinc oxide in sunscreen and tattoos, are also radiopaque. Generally, the large size and axillary location of such lesions suggest a benign etiology, but when faint, they sometimes are confused as suspicious. If there is uncertainty, careful skin cleansing will eliminate or greatly reduce their number.

■ Case 5–5

Calcification Morphology   Milk of calcium

Distribution of Calcifications   Diffuse/scattered

Clinical History   A 52-year-old woman presents for screening.

Physical Examination   Normal exam

Radiologic Findings

Mammography

Figure 5–5 Craniocaudal (CC) and mediolateral (ML) views. **(A)** CC magnification and **(B)** ML views. In the CC view, the calcifications are round or oval and slightly indistinct. In the ML view, the calcifications form curvilinear densities.

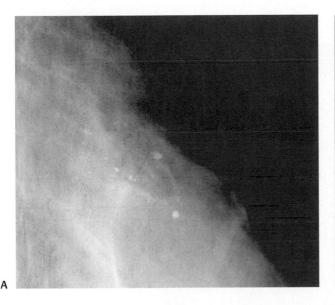 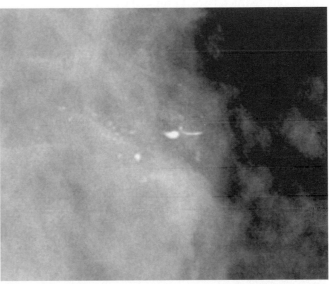

A   B

Management   BI-RADS category 2, benign finding

Pathologic Diagnosis

Benign

Milk of calcium

Pearls and Pitfalls

- Milk of calcium is precipitated calcium within microcysts. With a horizontal beam (ML or lateromedial [LM] views), the calcium layers at the bottom of the cysts and forms curvilinear or linear densities. With a vertical beam (CC view), the calcium forms ill-defined round densities.

■ Case 5–6

Calcification Morphology   Milk of calcium

Distribution of Calcifications   Diffuse/scattered

Clinical History   A 50-year-old woman presents for screening.

Physical Examination   Normal exam

Radiologic Findings

Mammography

Figure 5–6 Craniocaudal (CC) and mediolateral (ML) views. **(A)** Left CC magnification and **(B)** left ML magnification mammograms. In the inferior half of the breast, there are ill-defined oval and round calcifications on the CC view. However, on the ML view, these round calcifications are replaced by linear or semicircular "teacup" calcifications characteristic of milk of calcium.

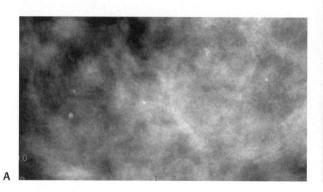
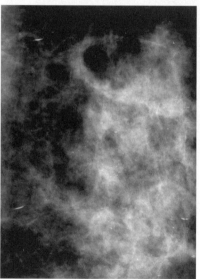

A   B

Management   BI-RADS category 2, benign finding

Pathologic Diagnosis

Benign

Milk of calcium

Pearls and Pitfalls

- This example demonstrates that manipulating the image with digital mammography is useful even after additional diagnostic views have been performed. Because these calcifications covered a broader area, the original magnified region was relatively large, and the smaller calcifications were difficult to evaluate even with the magnified views. Therefore, further manual digital magnification of the magnified views was useful in examining the entire area and characterizing the smaller calcifications.

■ Case 5–7

Calcification Morphology   Vascular

Clinical History   A 46-year-old woman presents for screening.

Physical Examination   Normal exam

Radiologic Findings

Mammography

Figure 5–7 Mediolateral oblique (MLO) views. **(A)** Left spot MLO magnification and **(B)** enlargement of mammogram. In the upper outer breast, there are a few long tortuous linear calcifications. These are consistent with vascular calcifications.

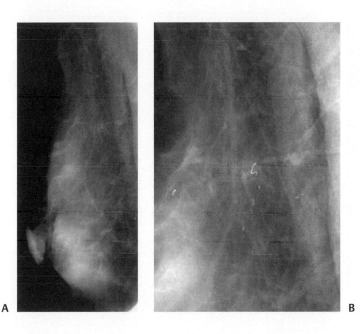

A   B

Management   BI-RADS category 2, benign finding

Pathologic Diagnosis

Benign

Vascular calcifications

Pearls and Pitfalls

- Vascular calcifications are generally long (>2 mm) and curvilinear. When they are small, they may be mistaken for DCIS. With suspected small vascular calcifications, a wider soft tissue window can be used to identify the blood vessels. Calcifications within the vessels can be followed using magnification.

■ Case 5–8

Calcification Morphology   Vascular

Clinical History   A 75-year-old woman presents for screening.

Physical Examination   Normal exam

Radiologic Findings

Mammography

Figure 5–8 Mediolateral oblique (MLO) and craniocaudal (CC) views. **(A)** Left MLO and **(B)** left CC mammograms. Curvilinear vascular calcifications are in the lateral and medial breast.

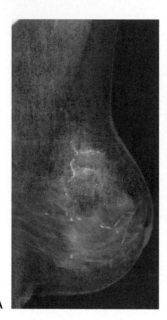
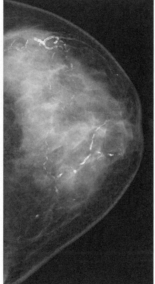

A   B

Management   BI-RADS category 2, benign finding

Pathologic Diagnosis

Benign

Atherosclerosis

Pearls and Pitfalls

- Arterial calcifications are curvilinear long depositions that are solid or tubular ("train track" calcifications). Occasionally, veins thrombose and form tortuous curvilinear calcifications, which are generally 2 to 3 times the thickness of the arteries.

■ Case 5–9

Calcification Morphology   Coarse/popcorn

Clinical History   A 56-year-old woman presents for screening.

Physical Examination   Normal exam

Radiologic Findings

Mammography

Figure 5–9 Mediolateral oblique (MLO) and craniocaudal (CC) views. **(A)** Left MLO mammogram, **(B)** left CC mammogram, and **(C)** enlargement of left MLO mammogram. There is a cluster of large, coarse calcifications at the 12 o'clock position.

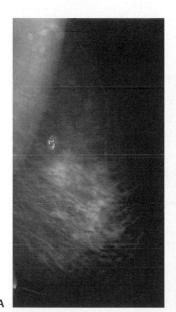 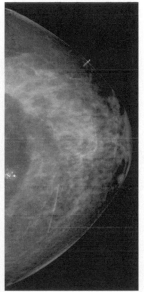 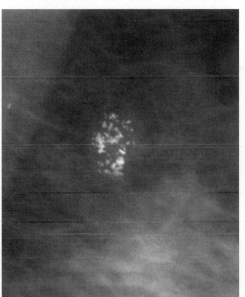

A   B   C

Management   BI-RADS category 2, benign finding

Pathologic Diagnosis

Benign

Fibroadenoma

Pearls and Pitfalls

- Fibroadenomas commonly present with large (>0.5 mm), irregularly shaped "popcorn" calcifications. Usually, these calcifications develop peripherally and extend centrally.

■ Case 5–10

Calcification Morphology   Dystrophic

Clinical History   An 84-year-old woman presents for screening.

Physical Examination   Normal exam

Radiologic Findings

Mammography

Figure 5–10 Mediolateral oblique (MLO) and craniocaudal (CC) views. **(A)** Right MLO, **(B)** right CC, **(C)** right enlarged CC posteriorly, and **(D)** right enlarged CC near nipple. In the upper outer quadrant, there is a cluster of large, coarse dystrophic calcifications consistent with a fibroadenoma **(C)**. These calcifications have been stable for more than 5 years. Vascular calcifications **(D)** are in the 3 o'clock position near the nipple.

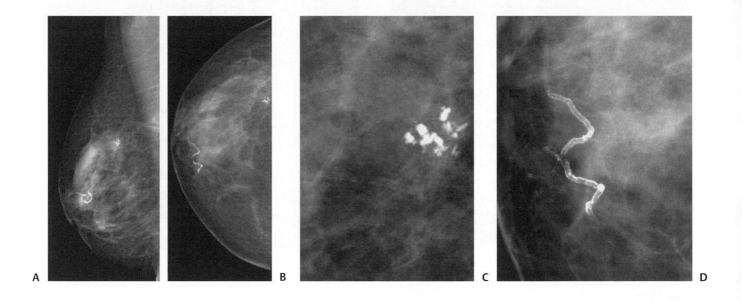

A   B   C   D

Management   BI-RADS category 2, benign finding

Pathologic Diagnosis

Benign

Fibroadenoma

Pearls and Pitfalls

- Fibroadenomas are the most common benign solid mass in women. About 25% of women autopsied have fibroadenomas. After menopause, fibroadenomas commonly involute, forming large, coarse calcifications.

■ Case 5–11

Calcification Morphology   Dystrophic

Clinical History   A 65-year-old woman presents for screening.

Physical Examination   Normal exam

Radiologic Findings

Mammography

Figure 5–11 Mediolateral oblique (MLO) and craniocaudal (CC) views. **(A)** Right MLO, **(B)** left MLO, **(C)** right CC, **(D)** left CC, and **(E)** left enlarged CC. There are scattered bilateral large, coarse dystrophic calcifications. These calcifications have been stable for more than 5 years.

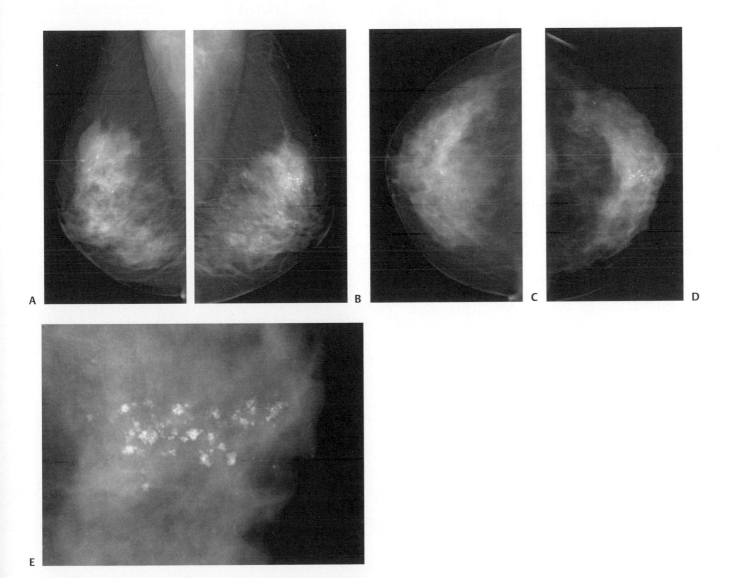

Management   BI-RADS category 2, benign finding

Pathologic Diagnosis

Benign

Dystrophic calcifications

Pearls and Pitfalls

• The large size and scattered distribution are characteristics of benign calcifications.

■ Case 5–12

Calcification Morphology   Dystrophic

Clinical History   An 86-year-old woman who had a lumpectomy 14 years ago presents for screening.

Physical Examination   Negative exam. No change is seen in left breast scar.

Radiologic Findings

Mammography

Figure 5–12 Mediolateral (ML) and craniocaudal (CC) views. **(A)** Left ML spot magnification and **(B)** left CC spot magnification views. There are multiple large round, lobular, and irregular calcifications.

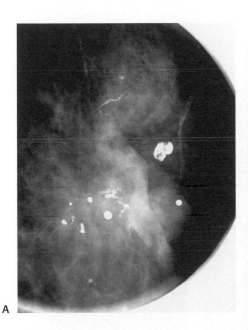 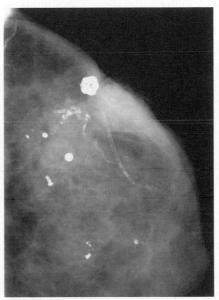

A   B

Management   BI-RADS category 2, benign finding

Pathologic Diagnosis

Benign

Dystrophic calcifications within scar

Pearls and Pitfalls

• These large calcifications are characteristic of fat necrosis and dystrophic calcifications within scar.

■ Case 5–13

Calcification Morphology   Dystrophic

Clinical History   A 74-year-old woman presents for screening. She had a right lumpectomy for breast cancer 14 years ago.

Physical Examination   Right breast: Normal exam. Well-healed lumpectomy scar. Left breast: Normal exam.

Radiologic Findings

Mammography

Figure 5–13 Mediolateral oblique (MLO) and craniocaudal (CC) views. **(A)** Right MLO (*without scar marker*), **(B)** right CC (*without scar marker*), **(C)** right MLO (*with scar marker*), and **(D)** right CC (*with scar marker*). There is a large single calcification at the 12:30 position. Current digital exam did not have scar marker. The previous digital exam scar markers clearly indicate that the calcification is related to the lumpectomy.

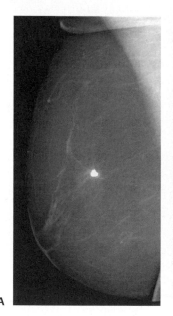
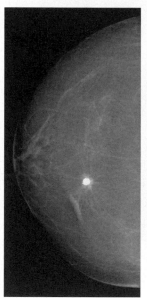
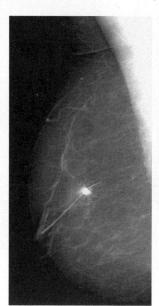
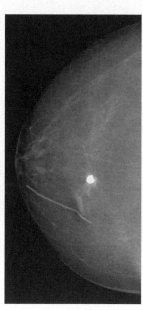

A   B–D

Management   BI-RADS category 2, benign finding

Pathologic Diagnosis

Benign

Dystrophic calcification

Pearls and Pitfalls

- The scar marker does not help in assessing the large single dystrophic calcification. However, the scar marker does help to clarify the etiology of the mild residual architectural distortion from the previous lumpectomy.

■ Case 5–14

Calcification Morphology   Dystrophic

Distribution of Calcifications   Regional

Clinical History   A 75-year-old woman who had a lumpectomy 9 years ago presents for screening. She notes new thickening at the lumpectomy site.

Physical Examination   Right breast: In the upper outer quadrant, there is firmness associated with the lumpectomy scar. Left breast: Normal exam.

Radiologic Findings

Mammography

Figure 5–14 Mediolateral oblique (MLO) and craniocaudal (CC) views. **(A)** Right MLO, **(B)** right CC, and **(C)** right ML spot magnification mammograms. There are numerous large, coarse, irregular calcifications in the right upper outer quadrant. Curvilinear vascular calcifications are also present.

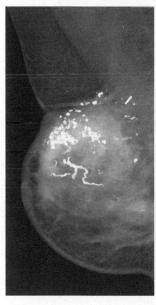 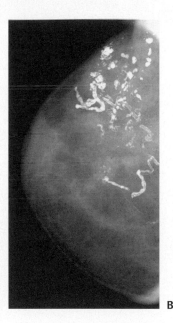 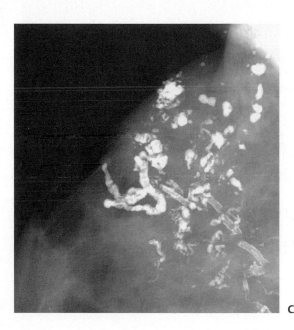

A   B   C

Ultrasonography

Figure 5–14 (**D**) Right radial and (**E**) right aradial sonographic images. Sonographic examination of the lumpectomy site demonstrated a hypoechoic irregular solid mass with architectural distortion, large shadowing calcifications, and skin thickening. These findings are nonspecific for scar or recurrence. (**F**) Bilateral breast three-dimensional contrast-enhanced dynamic magnetic resonance, subtraction image (2 minutes after contrast injection). Moderate early contrast enhancement of the lumpectomy scar is followed by a plateau in intensity. This kinetics pattern is non-specific, so biopsy was performed.

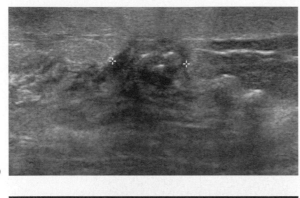
D

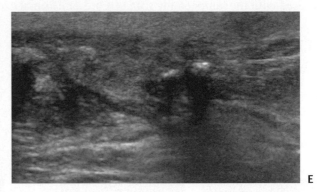
E

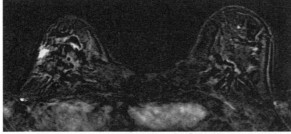
F

Management BI-RADS category 2, benign finding

Pathologic Diagnosis

Benign

Scar

Pearls and Pitfalls

- The large irregular calcifications are characteristic of dystrophic calcifications associated with scar.
- Although the calcifications are benign, the patient's lumpectomy site was further worked up because of her new clinical symptoms.

■ Case 5–15

Calcification Morphology   Eggshell/rim

Clinical History   A 50-year-old woman presents for screening.

Physical Examination   Normal exam

Radiologic Findings

Mammography

Figure 5–15 Mediolateral (ML) and craniocaudal (CC) views. **(A)** Right CC spot magnification mammogram and **(B)** right ML magnification mammogram. In the right upper inner breast, there is a single round eggshell calcification.

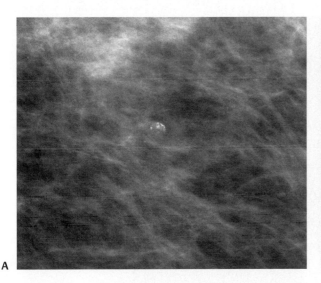
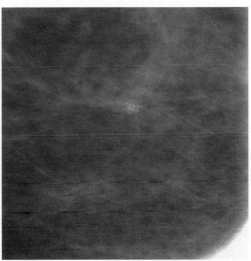

A   B

Management   BI-RADS category 2, benign finding

Pathologic Diagnosis

Benign

Cyst calcification

Pearls and Pitfalls

- Eggshell calcification indicates calcification of a cystic process—usually an oil cyst, rarely a fluid cyst. Digital mammography is much better in characterizing these cysts because a wider gray scale window can be used to demonstrate the nonuniformity of the calcification.

■ Case 5–16

Calcification Morphology   Round

Clinical History   A 55-year-old woman presents for screening.

Physical Examination   Normal exam

Radiologic Findings

Mammography

Figure 5–16 Mediolateral oblique (MLO) and craniocaudal (CC) views. **(A)** Right MLO and **(B)** right CC mammograms. At the 3 o'clock position, there is a single oval calcification.

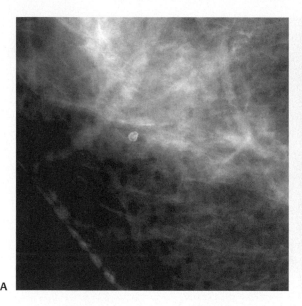
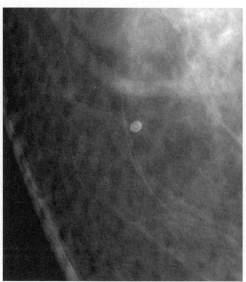

A   B

Management   BI-RADS category 2, benign finding

Pathologic Diagnosis

Benign

Fat necrosis

Pearls and Pitfalls

- Fat necrosis has many appearances; one of the most common is the oil cyst. The oil cyst is an oval or round calcified circumscribed mass.

■ Case 5–17

Calcification Morphology   Round

Distribution of Calcifications   Diffuse/scattered

Clinical History   A 73-year-old woman presents for screening.

Physical Examination   Normal exam

Radiologic Findings

Mammography

Figure 5–17 Mediolateral oblique (MLO) and craniocaudal (CC) views. **(A)** Right MLO, **(B)** left MLO, **(C)** right CC, **(D)** left CC, and **(E)** left CC enlarged. There are bilateral round and oval well-defined calcifications illustrative of oil cysts.

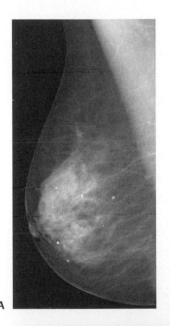
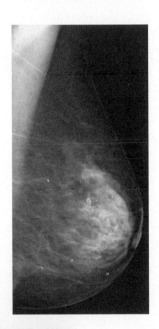
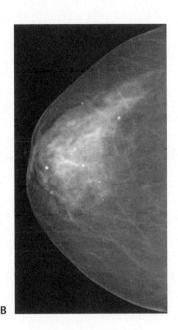
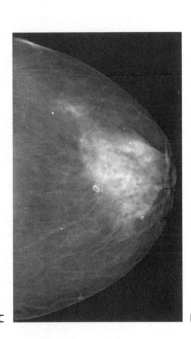

A   B   C   D

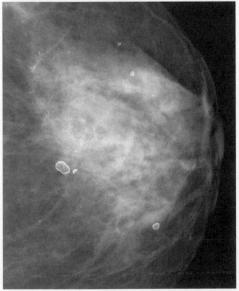

E

Management   BI-RADS category 2, benign finding

Pathologic Diagnosis

Benign

Fat necrosis

Pearls and Pitfalls

- Although oil cysts are a form of fat necrosis, commonly patients with oil cysts have no history of previous injury or surgery.

■ Case 5–18

Calcification Morphology   Punctate

Distribution of Calcifications   Diffuse/scattered

Clinical History   A 57-year-old woman presents for screening.

Physical Examination   Normal exam

Radiologic Findings

Mammography

Figure 5–18 Mediolateral (ML) and craniocaudal (CC) views. **(A)** Right ML magnification and **(B)** right CC magnification mammograms. There are scattered punctate and round calcifications throughout the breast.

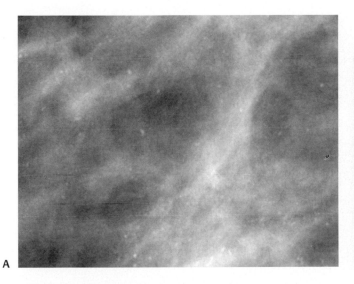
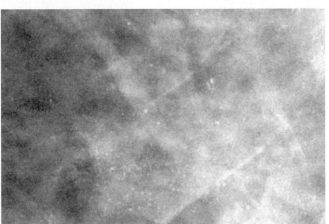

A   B

Management   BI-RADS category 2, benign finding

Pathologic Diagnosis

Benign

Sclerosing adenosis

Pearls and Pitfalls

- The round shape and scattered distribution are characteristic of sclerosing adenosis.

■ Case 5–19

Calcification Morphology   Round

Clinical History   A 57-year-old woman presents for screening.

Physical Examination   Normal exam

Radiologic Findings

Mammography

Figure 5–19 Mediolateral oblique (MLO) and craniocaudal (CC) views. **(A)** Right MLO, **(B)** right CC, **(C)** right MLO enlarged, and **(D)** right CC enlarged mammograms. There are scattered and clustered oval and round calcifications.

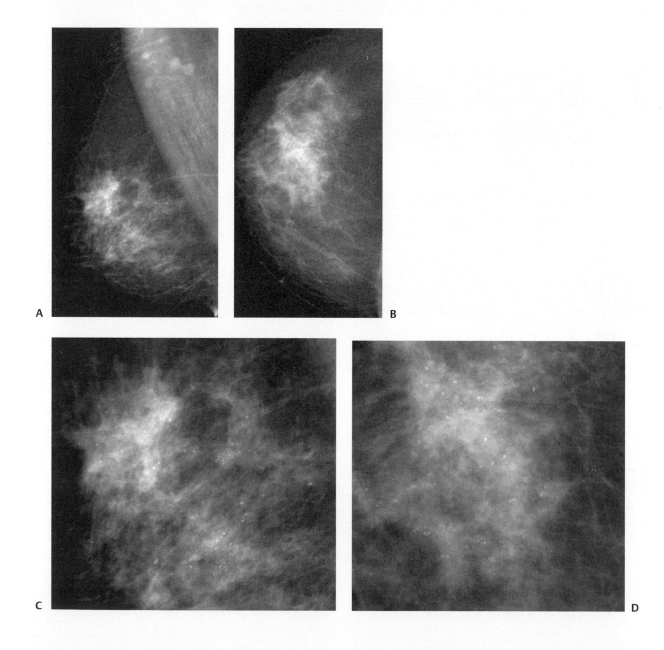

Management   BI-RADS category 2, benign finding

Pathologic Diagnosis

Benign

Calcifications in benign lobules

Pearls and Pitfalls

- These round calcifications are characteristic of those within lobules.

■ Case 5–20

Calcification Morphology   Punctate

Distribution of Calcifications   Grouped/clustered

Clinical History   A 47-year-old woman presents for screening.

Physical Examination   Normal exam

Radiologic Findings

Mammography

Figure 5–20 Mediolateral oblique (MLO) and craniocaudal (CC) views. **(A)** Right MLO and **(B)** right CC mammograms. There is a cluster of punctate calcifications (circled) that has been stable for at least 3 years.

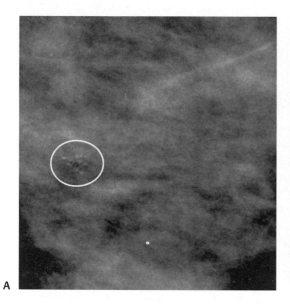
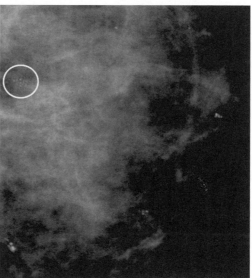

A   B

Management   BI-RADS category 2, benign finding

Pathologic Diagnosis

Benign

Calcifications in benign lobules

Pearls and Pitfalls

- This case illustrates that digital mammography is useful in avoiding unnecessary recalls. Because these calcifications are small, they are difficult to characterize on the screening images. They were electronically magnified and proved to be unchanged upon comparison with electronically magnified digital screen images produced 3 years earlier.

■ Case 5–21

Calcification Morphology Large, rodlike

Distribution of Calcifications Diffuse/scattered

Clinical History A 78-year-old woman presents for screening.

Physical Examination Normal exam

Radiologic Findings

Mammography

Figure 5–21 Mediolateral oblique (MLO) and craniocaudal (CC) views. **(A)** Right MLO, **(B)** right CC, and **(C)** right enlarged CC mammograms. There are diffuse, scattered, thick linear calcifications that are oriented toward the nipple.

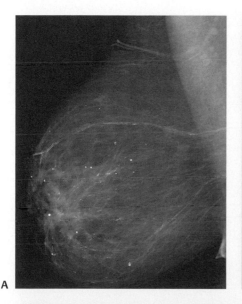
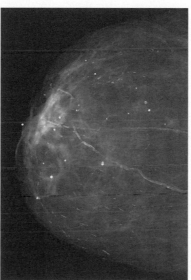

A
B

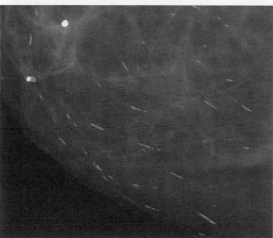

C

Management BI-RADS category 2, benign finding

Pathologic Diagnosis

Benign

Plasma cell mastitis

Pearls and Pitfalls

- This benign pattern of large linear or rodlike calcifications (also labeled secretory calcifications) oriented toward the nipple are characteristic of plasma cell mastitis. Microscopically, the calcifications are within dilated ducts, which also contain inflammatory cells and necrotic debris. Periductal inflammation may also be present. These patients are asymptomatic and do not have an increased risk of cancer.

■ Case 5–22

Calcification Morphology   Punctate

Clinical History   A 57-year-old woman presents for screening.

Physical Examination   Normal exam

Radiologic Findings

Mammography

Figure 5–22 Left mediolateral oblique magnification mammogram. There is a cluster of round and punctate calcifications (*circled*) next to the chest wall.

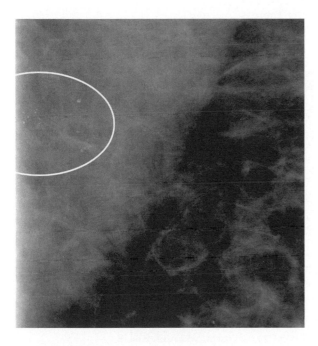

Management   BI-RADS category 3, probably benign. Short-interval follow-up.

Pathologic Diagnosis

Benign

Calcifications in benign lobules

Pearls and Pitfalls

- Punctate calcifications are differentiated from round calcifications by size. Punctate calcifications are less than 0.5 mm, and round calcifications are larger.

■ Case 5–23

Calcification Morphology   Punctate

Distribution of Calcifications   Grouped/clustered

Clinical History   A 64-year-old woman has a new cluster of calcifications.

Physical Examination   Normal exam

Radiologic Findings

Mammography

Figure 5–23 Mediolateral oblique (MLO) and craniocaudal (CC) views. **(A)** Left MLO spot magnification and **(B)** left CC spot magnification mammograms. There is a cluster of punctate calcifications in the upper outer quadrant.

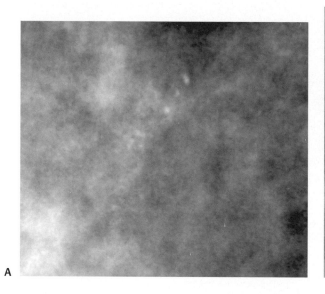
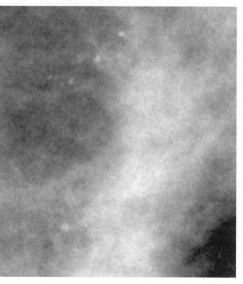

A   B

Management   BI-RADS category 3, probably benign. Short-interval follow-up.

Pathologic Diagnosis

Benign

Sclerosing adenosis

Pearls and Pitfalls

- Adenosis reflects lobular disease, including lobular hyperplasia and sclerosing adenosis. The mammographic findings include diffuse, scattered 3- to 5-mm ill-defined nodules with or without scattered round calcifications.

■ Case 5–24

Calcification Morphology   Punctate

Distribution of Calcifications   Grouped/clustered

Clinical History   A 37-year-old woman with strong family history of breast cancer presents for a baseline exam.

Physical Examination   Normal exam

Radiologic Findings

Mammography

Figure 5–24 Lateromedial (LM) and craniocaudal (CC) views. **(A)** Left LM magnification and **(B)** left CC magnification mammograms. A cluster of punctate calcifications is seen in the upper outer quadrant.

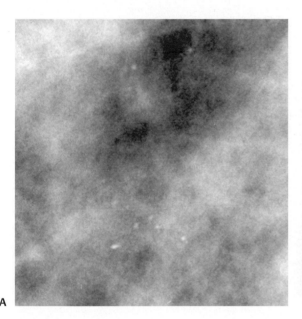
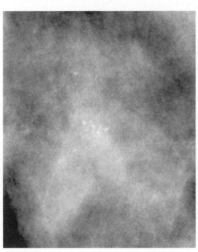

A   B

Management   BI-RADS category 3, probably benign. Short-interval follow-up.

Pathologic Diagnosis

Benign

Calcifications in benign lobules

Pearls and Pitfalls

- Although punctate calcifications are usually benign, they should be followed closely because they may reflect early findings of DCIS.

■ Case 5–25

Calcification Morphology   Punctate

Distribution of Calcifications   Grouped/clustered

Clinical History   A 61-year-old woman with known left breast cancer presents for screening. The patient has a new cluster of right punctate calcifications.

Physical Examination   Right breast: Normal exam.

Radiologic Findings

Mammography

Figure 5–25 Mediolateral (ML) and craniocaudal (CC) views. **(A)** Right ML magnification and **(B)** right CC magnification mammograms. There is a cluster of punctate calcifications in the right upper outer quadrant.

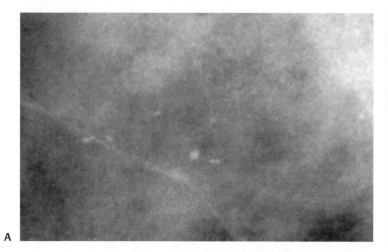
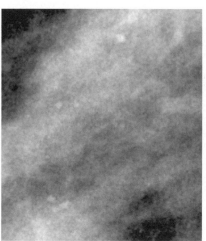

Management   BI-RADS category 3, probably benign. Short-interval follow-up.

Pathologic Diagnosis

Benign

Benign fibrosis and microcysts

Pearls and Pitfalls

- These calcifications appear to be benign because, with digital manual magnification, the shapes are round. However, because the patient was being evaluated for left breast cancer treatment, she elected to biopsy these calcifications.

■ Case 5–26

Calcification Morphology   Punctate

Distribution of Calcifications   Grouped/clustered

Clinical History   A 42-year-old woman with right increasing calcifications presents for screening.

Physical Examination   Bilateral breasts: Normal exam.

Radiologic Findings

Mammography

Figure 5–26 Mediolateral oblique (MLO) and craniocaudal (CC) views. **(A)** Right MLO magnification and **(B)** right CC magnification mammograms. In the subareolar area, there is a cluster of punctate and round calcifications. There is more overlap of calcifications in the MLO view, so their shape is less clear.

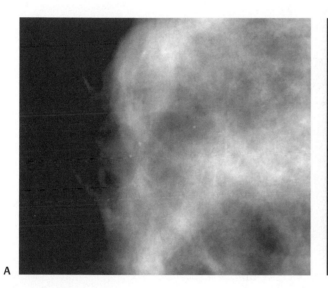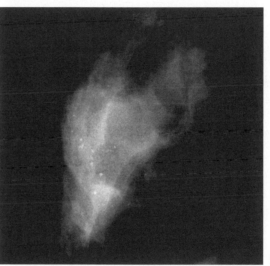

A   B

Management   BI-RADS category 4, suspicious. Biopsy should be considered.

Pathologic Diagnosis

Benign

Calcifications in benign fibrocystic tissue

Pearls and Pitfalls

- Although punctate and round calcifications are normally considered probably benign, because these calcifications were increasing in number, they were considered suspicious.

■ Case 5–27

Calcification Morphology   Punctate

Distribution of Calcifications   Grouped/clustered

Clinical History   A 50-year-old woman presents for screening.

Physical Examination   Normal exam

Radiologic Findings

Mammography

Figure 5–27 Mediolateral oblique (MLO) and craniocaudal (CC) views. **(A)** Right CC magnification and **(B)** right MLO magnification mammograms. There is a new cluster of punctate calcifications in the upper outer quadrant. These calcifications may be slightly more suspicious because they appear to be slightly heterogeneous in size.

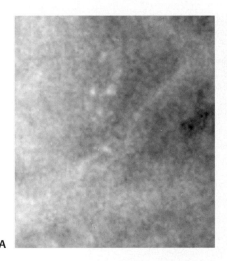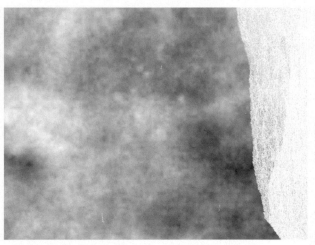

A

Management   BI-RADS category 3, probably benign. Short-interval follow-up.

Pathologic Diagnosis

Benign

Atypical ductal hyperplasia (ADH)

Pearls and Pitfalls

- DCIS differs from ADH only in the size of the affected area. ADH is defined by abnormal proliferation (1) confined to only a part of the terminal duct lobular unit (TDLU), (2) involving no more than two TDLUs, and (3) not greater than 2 mm. If this proliferation is larger than these parameters, then the lesion is DCIS. If only ADH is identified on a biopsy sample, then excision is necessary to adequately exclude neoplasia.

Case 5–28

Calcification Morphology   Punctate

Distribution of Calcifications   Grouped/clustered

Clinical History   An 81-year-old woman presents for screening.

Physical Examination   Bilateral breasts: Normal exam.

Radiologic Findings

Mammography

Figure 5–28 Right mediolateral magnification mammogram. A cluster of punctate calcifications (*circled*) are at the 3 o'clock position of the breast. Although these were punctate, they were assessed as suspicious because they were increasing in number since the previous year.

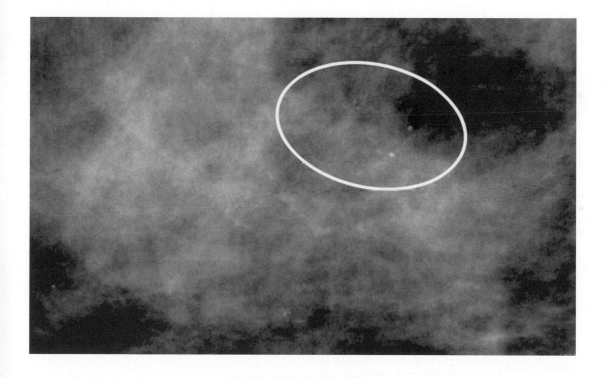

Management   BI-RADS category 4, suspicious. Biopsy should be considered.

Pathologic Diagnosis

Malignant

Invasive ductal carcinoma

Pearls and Pitfalls

- Fortunately, this patient's malignancy was very small, only 0.6 cm in diameter.

■ Case 5–29

Calcification Morphology   Punctate

Distribution of Calcifications   Grouped/clustered

Clinical History   A 54-year-old woman with increasing left breast calcifications presents for screening.

Physical Examination   Normal exam

Radiologic Findings

Mammography

Figure 5–29 Mediolateral oblique (MLO). **(A)** Left MLO magnification and **(B)** enlargement of calcifications in **(A)**. A cluster of punctate calcifications are in the upper outer quadrant.

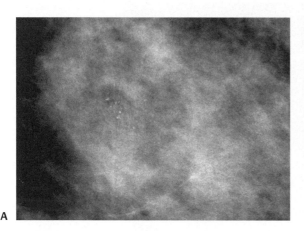
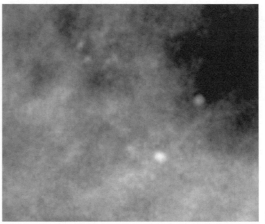

A   B

Management   BI-RADS category 4, suspicious. Biopsy should be considered.

Pathologic Diagnosis

Malignant

Invasive ductal carcinoma with a predominantly intraductal component

Comments on Histology   0.2 cm invasive tumor without significant intraductal component

Pearls and Pitfalls

- Although round calcifications are generally due to benign lobular calcifications, ductal neoplasms may spread into the lobules, producing round calcifications.

■ Case 5–30

Calcification Morphology   Amorphous/indistinct

Distribution of Calcifications   Grouped/clustered

Clinical History   A 76-year-old woman presents for screening.

Physical Examination   Normal exam

Radiologic Findings

Mammography

Figure 5–30 Lateromedial (LM) and exaggerated craniocaudal (XCCL) views. **(A)** Left LM magnification and **(B)** XCCL magnification mammograms. There is a cluster of amorphous calcifications in the upper outer quadrant.

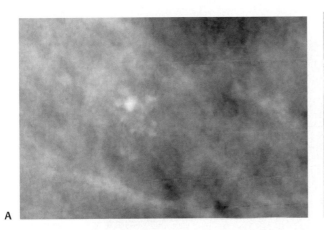
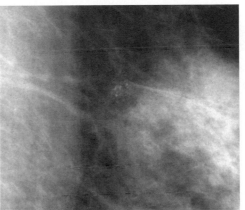

A   B

Management   BI-RADS category 4, suspicious. Biopsy should be considered.

Pathologic Diagnosis

Benign

ADH

Pearls and Pitfalls

- Women with ADH have a 5 times greater risk for breast malignancy than the normal population.

■ Case 5–31

Calcification Morphology   Amorphous/indistinct

Clinical History   A 71-year-old woman who had right mixed invasive ductal and lobular cancer 7 years ago presents for screening.

Physical Examination   Right breast: Normal scar in upper outer quadrant.

Radiologic Findings

Mammography

Figure 5–31 Mediolateral oblique (MLO) and craniocaudal (CC) views. **(A)** Right MLO magnification, **(B)** right CC magnification, and **(C)** right CC magnification mammograms. In the upper outer quadrant, there are new segmentally distributed punctate and amorphous calcifications that are arranged in a linear pattern (*arrows*).

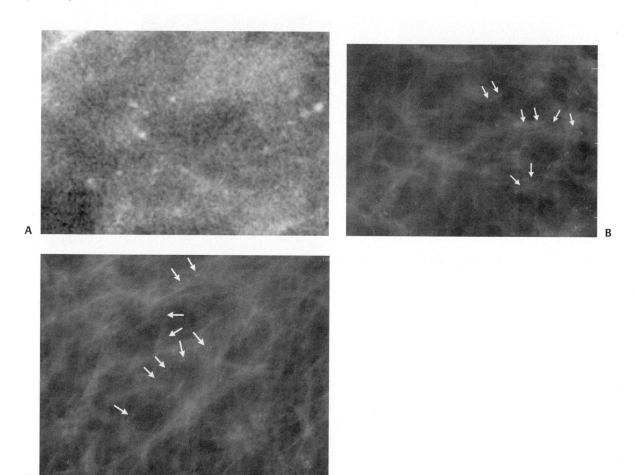

Management   BI-RADS category 4, suspicious. Biopsy should be considered.

Pathologic Diagnosis

Malignant

DCIS

Pearls and Pitfalls

- Although the linear pattern strongly suggests DCIS, this pattern is difficult to appreciate because the calcifications are thinly spread over a large area of the breast. In this case, a large magnification compression panel is better than a small spot magnification paddle, as these calcifications may appear scattered or may be missed by the small field of view.

■ Case 5–32

Calcification Morphology Amorphous/indistinct

Distribution of Calcifications Grouped/clustered

Clinical History A 49-year-old woman presents for screening.

Physical Examination Bilateral breasts: Normal exam.

Radiologic Findings

Mammography

Figure 5–32 Mediolateral (ML) and craniocaudal (CC) views. **(A)** Right ML magnification and **(B)** right CC magnification mammograms. There is a large cluster of new amorphous calcifications in the upper outer quadrant (*circled*). **(C)** Right ML magnification and **(D)** right CC magnification mammograms. There were inadequate surgical margins after the initial excision, so repeat mammograms were performed. Unfortunately, amorphous calcifications are still present in the region of the site of excision (*circled*). Final surgical excision removed all of the calcifications. The specimen was a mixture of DCIS and ADH.

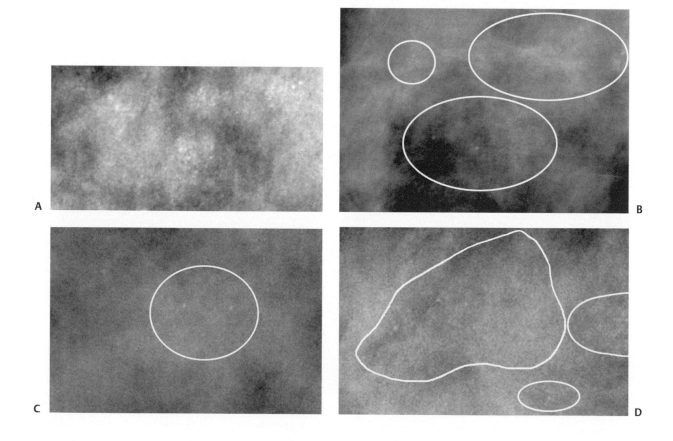

Management   BI-RADS Category 4, suspicious. Biopsy should be considered.

Pathologic Diagnosis

Malignant

DCIS

Pearls and Pitfalls

- Amorphous calcifications have been found to represent malignancy in ~20% of cases. In the malignant cases, the histology is either invasive malignancy or DCIS.

■ Case 5–33

Calcification Morphology   Amorphous/indistinct

Distribution of Calcifications   Grouped/clustered

Clinical History   A 67-year-old woman presents for screening.

Physical Examination   Bilateral breasts: Normal exam.

Radiologic Findings

Mammography

Figure 5–33 Left mediolateral oblique magnification mammogram. There is a new cluster of amorphous calcifications in the central breast.

Management   BI-RADS category 4, suspicious. Biopsy should be considered.

Pathologic Diagnosis

Malignant

DCIS

Pearls and Pitfalls

- Amorphous calcifications are difficult to identify prospectively. They have poor conspicuity and are particularly difficult to identify in heterogeneous or extremely dense breasts.

■ Case 5–34

Calcification Morphology   Coarse heterogeneous

Distribution of Calcifications   Grouped/clustered

Clinical History   A 50-year-old woman who had a left lumpectomy and radiation therapy 3 years ago presents for screening.

Physical Examination   Left breast: Normal lumpectomy scar.

Radiologic Findings

Mammography

Figure 5–34 Mediolateral oblique (MLO) and craniocaudal (CC) views. **(A)** Left MLO magnification and **(B)** left CC magnification mammograms. There is a new cluster of coarse heterogeneous calcifications (*circled*) in the lumpectomy scar.

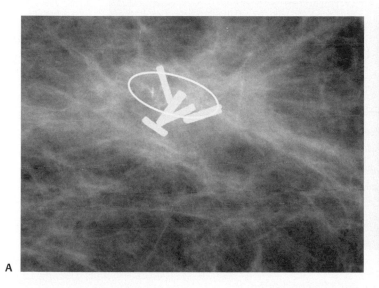
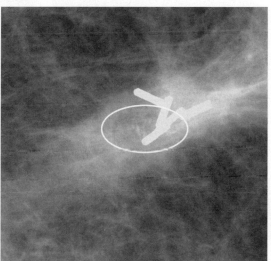

A   B

Management   BI-RADS category 4, suspicious. Biopsy should be considered.

Pathologic Diagnosis

Benign

Fat necrosis

Pearls and Pitfalls

- The recurrence rate for lumpectomy and radiation therapy is ~1% per year for a total of ~10 to 15% for 10 years. Although coarse heterogeneous calcifications are commonly due to dystrophic changes, they should be biopsied because of the high risk of recurrence.

■ Case 5–35

Calcification Morphology   Coarse heterogeneous

Distribution of Calcifications   Grouped/clustered

Clinical History   A 42-year-old woman presents for screening.

Physical Examination   Bilateral breasts: Normal exam.

Radiologic Findings

Mammography

Figure 5–35 Mediolateral (ML) and craniocaudal (CC) views. **(A)** Left ML magnification and **(B)** left CC magnification mammograms. There is a new cluster of coarse heterogeneous calcifications in the upper outer quadrant.

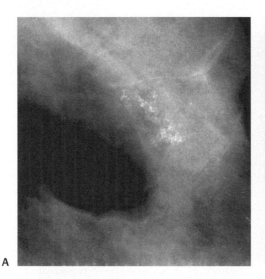
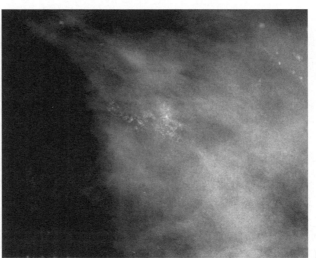

A   B

Management   BI-RADS category 4, suspicious. Biopsy should be considered.

Pathologic Diagnosis

Benign

Benign fibrocystic tissue

Pearls and Pitfalls

- Coarse heterogeneous calcifications are irregular, conspicuous, and generally larger than 0.5 mm. However, they are smaller than dystrophic calcifications and should be biopsied if they are new or increasing.

■ Case 5–36

Calcification Morphology   Coarse heterogeneous

Distribution of Calcifications   Grouped/clustered

Clinical History   A 69-year-old woman presents for screening.

Physical Examination   Bilateral breasts: Normal exam.

Radiologic Findings

Mammography

Figure 5–36   Lateromedial (LM) and craniocaudal (CC) views. **(A)** Left LM magnification and **(B)** left CC magnification mammograms. There is a small cluster of coarse heterogeneous calcifications in the upper outer quadrant.

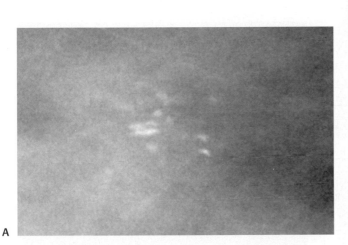 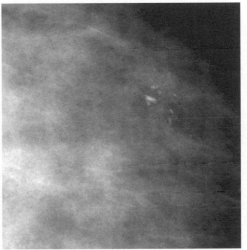

A   B

Management   BI-RADS category 4, suspicious. Biopsy should be considered.

Pathologic Diagnosis

Benign

Fibroadenoma

Pearls and Pitfalls

- Benign entities that produce coarse heterogeneous calcifications include fibroadenoma, fibrosis, and dystrophic change from trauma.

■ Case 5–37

Calcification Morphology   Coarse heterogeneous

Distribution of Calcifications   Grouped/clustered

Clinical History   A 49-year-old woman presents for screening.

Physical Examination   Bilateral breasts: Normal exam.

Radiologic Findings

Mammography

Figure 5–37 Mediolateral (ML) and craniocaudal (CC) views. **(A)** Right spot ML, **(B)** right spot CC, and **(C)** right enlarged ML mammograms. There is a cluster of coarse heterogeneous calcifications at the 12 o'clock position.

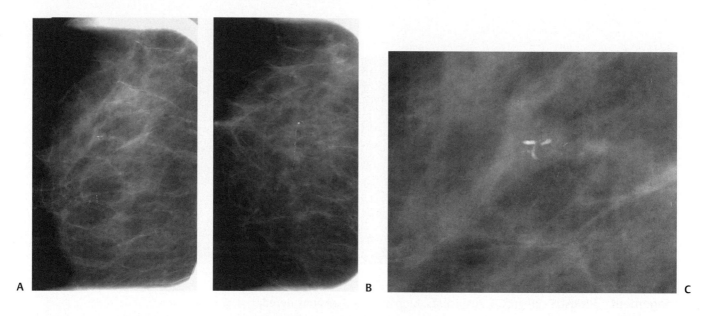

A

B

C

Management   BI-RADS category 4, suspicious. Biopsy should be considered.

Pathologic Diagnosis

Benign

Papilloma with sclerosis

Pearls and Pitfalls

- Coarse heterogeneous calcifications tend to be easily visible without magnification.

■ Case 5–38

Calcification Morphology   Coarse heterogeneous

Distribution of Calcifications   Segmental

Clinical History   A 68-year-old woman presents with new left breast calcifications.

Physical Examination   Left breast: Generalized firmness in the upper outer quadrant.

Radiologic Findings

Mammography

Figure 5–38 Craniocaudal (CC) and mediolateral (ML) views. **(A)** Left CC magnification and **(B)** left ML magnification mammograms. In the upper outer quadrant, there are coarse heterogeneous calcifications in a segmental distribution. Within this segment, the calcifications appear to follow a linear pattern.

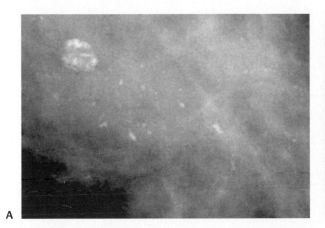
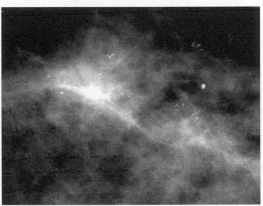

A   B

Management   BI-RADS category 4, suspicious. Biopsy should be considered.

Pathologic Diagnosis

Malignant

DCIS

Pearls and Pitfalls

- The segmental distribution and linear pattern of the coarse heterogeneous calcifications suggests the presence of DCIS. This assessment should be either category 4C or 5 because of the distribution of the calcifications.

■ Case 5–39

Calcification Morphology   Fine pleomorphic

Distribution of Calcifications   Grouped/clustered

Clinical History   A 54-year-old woman presents with new right calcifications.

Physical Examination   Normal exam

Radiologic Findings

Mammography

Figure 5–39 Right mediolateral oblique mammogram. In the lower inner quadrant, there is a cluster of fine pleomorphic calcifications.

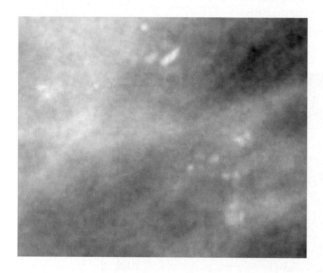

Management   BI-RADS category 4, suspicious. Biopsy should be considered.

Pathologic Diagnosis

Benign

Benign microcysts, stromal fibrosis

Pearls and Pitfalls

- Fine pleomorphic calcifications are less than 0.5 mm and are generally intermediate to high in suspiciousness.

■ Case 5–40

Calcification Morphology   Fine pleomorphic

Distribution of Calcifications   Grouped/clustered

Clinical History   A 67-year-old woman presents for screening.

Physical Examination   Normal exam

Radiologic Findings

Mammography

Figure 5–40   Mediolateral oblique (MLO) and craniocaudal (CC) views. **(A)** Right MLO magnification and **(B)** right CC magnification mammograms. There is a cluster of fine pleomorphic calcifications (*arrow*) at the 12 o'clock position.

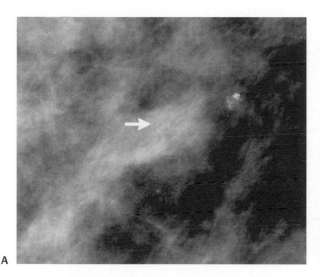
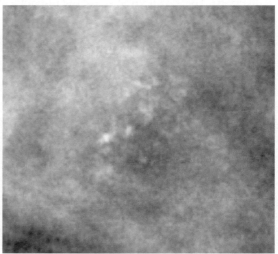

A   B

Management   BI-RADS category 4, suspicious. Biopsy should be considered.

Pathologic Diagnosis

Benign

Fibrocystic changes

Comments on Histology   Calcifications in benign ducts and microcysts

Pearls and Pitfalls

- Benign causes for pleomorphic calcifications include fibrocystic change and sclerosing adenosis.

■ Case 5–41

Calcification Morphology   Fine pleomorphic

Distribution of Calcifications   Grouped/clustered

Clinical History   A 47-year-old woman presents for a 6-month follow-up for left upper quadrant asymmetry.

Physical Examination   Normal exam

Radiologic Findings

Mammography

Figure 5–41 Mediolateral oblique (MLO) and exaggerated craniocaudal (XCCL) views. **(A)** Left MLO magnification and **(B)** left XCCL magnification mammograms. In the posterior half depth of the upper outer quadrant, there is a cluster of fine pleomorphic calcifications. These were new since the previous exam.

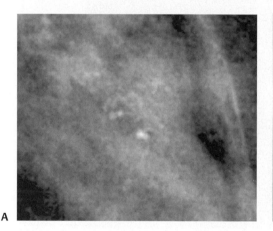 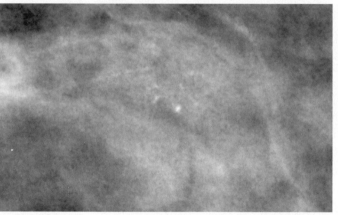

A   B

Management   BI-RADS category 4, suspicious. Biopsy should be considered.

Pathologic Diagnosis

Benign

Fibrocystic changes

Comments on Histology   Calcifications in benign microcysts and ducts

Pearls and Pitfalls

- Fine pleomorphic calcifications are more visible than amorphous calcifications, which allows identification of the nonuniform shapes of the calcifications.

■ Case 5–42

Calcification Morphology   Fine pleomorphic

Distribution of Calcifications   Grouped/clustered

Clinical History   A 59-year-old woman presents for screening.

Physical Examination   Normal exam

Radiologic Findings

Mammography

Figure 5–42 Mediolateral (ML) and craniocaudal (CC) views. **(A)** Right ML magnification and **(B)** CC magnification mammograms. At the 12 o'clock position, there is a cluster of fine pleomorphic calcifications.

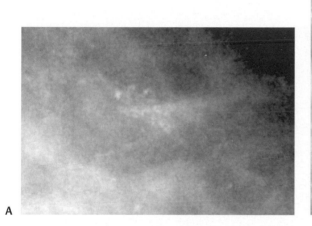
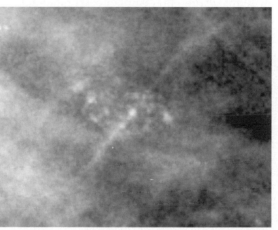

A   B

Management   BI-RADS category 4, suspicious. Biopsy should be considered.

Pathologic Diagnosis

Benign

ADH

Pearls and Pitfalls

- When ADH is identified by percutaneous biopsy, malignancy is found in up to 25% of patients who have these lesions excised.

■ Case 5–43

Calcification Morphology   Fine pleomorphic

Distribution of Calcifications   Grouped/clustered

Clinical History   A 48-year-old woman presents for screening.

Physical Examination   Normal exam

Radiologic Findings

Mammography

Figure 5–43 Mediolateral (ML) and craniocaudal (CC) views. **(A)** Right ML magnification, **(B)** right CC magnification, **(C)** right digital enlargement of ML magnification, **(D)** white and black inversion of **(C)**, **(E)** right digital enlargement of CC magnification, and **(F)** white and black inversion of **(E)**. There is a cluster of fine pleomorphic calcifications (*arrow*) in the upper outer quadrant.

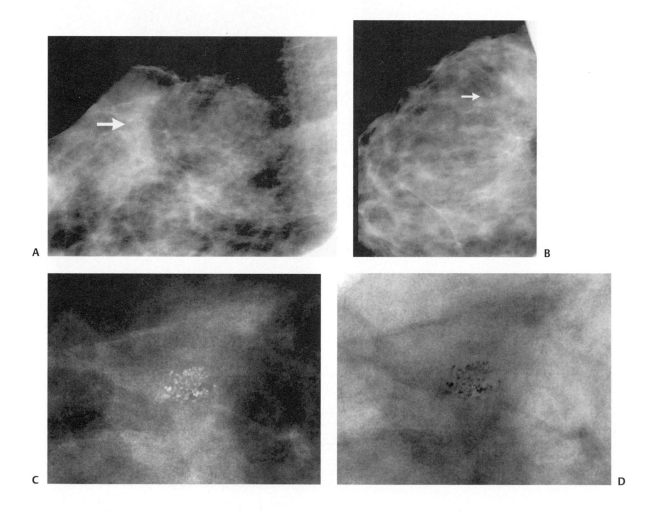

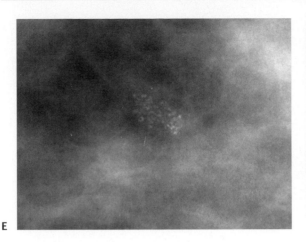

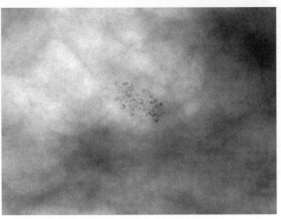

E

F

Management   BI-RADS category 4, suspicious. Biopsy should be considered.

Pathologic Diagnosis

Benign

ADH

Pearls and Pitfalls

- These images demonstrate the usefulness of digitally enlarging areas of interest in a mammogram. Although magnification views improve visualization of calcifications, digital enlargement of the calcifications from these views further clarifies the appearance of this lesion.
- Occasionally, the shapes of calcifications are better identified with inverting the white-and-black presentation mode.

■ Case 5–44

Calcification Morphology   Fine pleomorphic

Distribution of Calcifications   Grouped/clustered

Clinical History   A 57-year-old woman presents for screening.

Physical Examination   Normal exam

Radiologic Findings

Mammography

Figure 5–44 Craniocaudal (CC) and mediolateral (ML) views. **(A)** Right CC magnification and **(B)** right ML magnification mammograms. At the 7 o'clock position, there is a new cluster of fine pleomorphic calcifications.

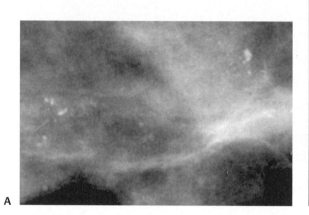
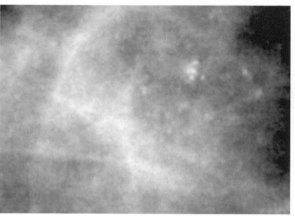

A   B

Management   BI-RADS category 4, suspicious. Biopsy should be considered.

Pathologic Diagnosis

Benign

ADH

Pearls and Pitfalls

- When the cluster of fine pleomorphic calcifications is small (<1 cm³), there are numerous histologies that would be concordant with a core biopsy as long as calcifications are within the specimen. For example, in this case, besides malignancy and ADH, fibrocystic calcifications, fibroadenomatous hyperplasia, and dystrophic change would all be acceptable correlates.

■ Case 5–45

Calcification Morphology   Fine pleomorphic

Distribution of Calcifications   Grouped/clustered

Clinical History   An 84-year-old woman presents for screening.

Physical Examination   Left breast: Normal exam.

Radiologic Findings

Mammography

Figure 5–45 Lateromedial (LM) and craniocaudal (CC) views. **(A)** Left LM magnification and **(B)** left CC magnification mammograms. There is a cluster of fine pleomorphic calcifications in the upper outer quadrant.

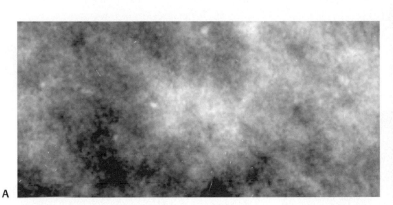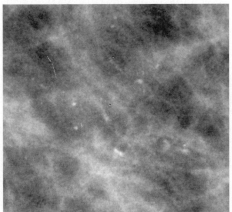

Management   BI-RADS category 4, suspicious. Biopsy should be considered.

Pathologic Diagnosis

Malignant

DCIS

Pearls and Pitfalls

- These fine pleomorphic calcifications are oriented in a linear and branching pattern, so they are more suspicious for DCIS.

■ Case 5–46

Calcification Morphology   Fine pleomorphic

Distribution of Calcifications   Segmental

Clinical History   A 64-year-old woman is 1-year status post–right lumpectomy and x-ray therapy for invasive ductal cancer. She now has new left breast calcifications.

Physical Examination   Left breast: Normal exam. Right breast: Healing lumpectomy scar.

Radiologic Findings

Mammography

Figure 5–46 Mediolateral (ML) and craniocaudal (CC) views. **(A)** Left ML magnification, **(B)** left CC magnification, **(C)** and **(D)** are enlarged portions of **(B)** mammograms. In the upper outer quadrant of the left breast, there is a segmental distribution of multiple clusters of fine pleomorphic calcifications (*circled*).

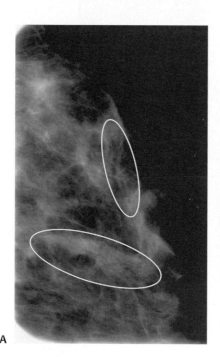
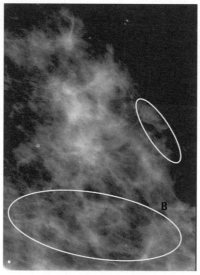
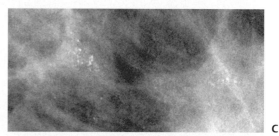
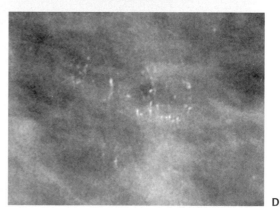

Management   BI-RADS category 4, suspicious. Biopsy should be considered.

Pathologic Diagnosis

Malignant

DCIS

Pearls and Pitfalls

- The segmental distribution of these fine pleomorphic calcifications elevates their suspicious appearance to a BI-RADS Category 4C.

■ Case 5–47

Calcification Morphology   Fine pleomorphic

Distribution of Calcifications   Grouped/clustered

Clinical History   An 81-year-old woman presents for screening.

Physical Examination   Normal exam

Radiologic Findings

Mammography

Figure 5–47 Left mediolateral magnification mammogram. There is a cluster of fine pleomorphic calcifications in the posterior aspect of the breast.

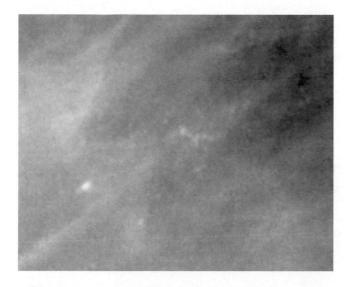

Management   BI-RADS category 4, suspicious. Biopsy should be considered.

Pathologic Diagnosis

Malignant

DCIS

Pearls and Pitfalls

- The smaller size and lack of either a linear or segmental distribution result in assessing these calcifications as a BI-RADS category 4B.

■ Case 5–48

Calcification Morphology   Fine pleomorphic

Distribution of Calcifications   Grouped/clustered

Clinical History   A 74–year-old woman who had a left lumpectomy and radiation therapy for breast cancer 3 years ago presents for screening.

Physical Examination   Right breast: Normal exam. Left breast: Normal, well-healed scar.

Radiologic Findings

Mammography

Figure 5–48 Mediolateral (ML), craniocaudal (CC) and mediolateral oblique (MLO) views. **(A)** Right ML magnification, **(B)** right ML magnification with white and black inverted, **(C)** right CC magnification, and **(D)** right CC magnification with white and black inverted mammograms. There is a cluster of fine pleomorphic calcifications in the upper outer quadrant. **(B)** and **(D)** demonstrate the appearance of the fine pleomorphic calcifications with white and black inversion. **(E)** Right MLO and **(F)** right CC mammograms. These views demonstrate electronic marking of the screening images to guide the patient's further workup.

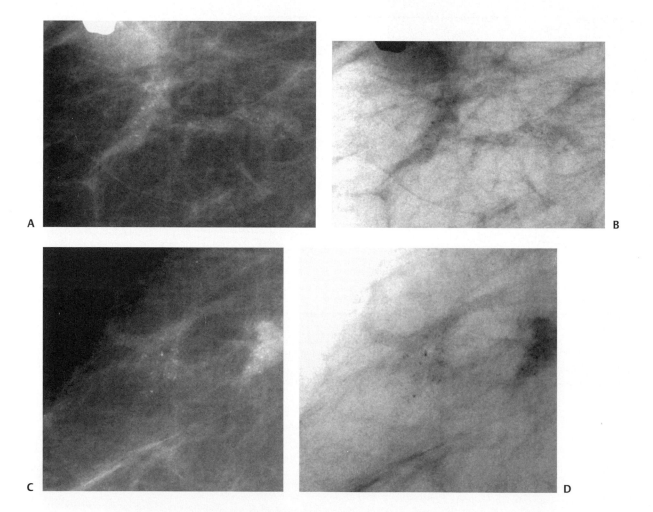

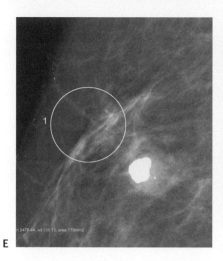

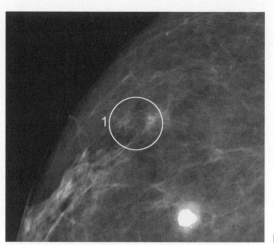

E
F

Management   BI-RADS category 4, suspicious. Biopsy should be considered.

Pathologic Diagnosis

Malignant

DCIS

Pearls and Pitfalls

- When a screening mammogram patient is being called back for additional views, the images can be electronically marked to guide the subsequent markup. These additional views may be permanently saved or discarded from the patient's permanent digital file.

■ Case 5–49

Calcification Morphology   Fine pleomorphic

Distribution of Calcifications   Grouped/clustered

Clinical History   A 42-year-old woman presents with a right breast lump.

Physical Examination   Right breast: Lump in upper outer quadrant.

Radiologic Findings

Mammography

Figure 5–49 Mediolateral oblique (MLO) and craniocaudal (CC) views. **(A)** Right MLO magnification and **(B)** right CC magnification mammograms. In the upper outer quadrant, there is a cluster of fine pleomorphic calcifications that corresponds to the palpable lump.

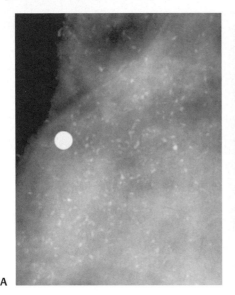
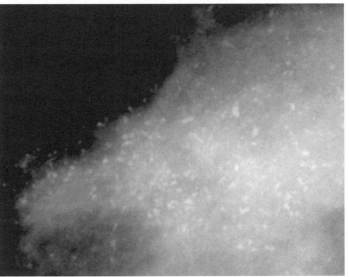

A   B

Management   BI-RADS category 5, highly suggestive of malignancy

Pathologic Diagnosis

Malignant

DCIS

Pearls and Pitfalls

- This case demonstrates a classic appearance of fine pleomorphic calcifications in a linear branching distribution. The calcifications are irregular and granular or rounded in shape. They form within pockets of necrotic DCIS. The patient had high-grade DCIS.

■ Case 5–50

Calcification Morphology   Fine pleomorphic

Distribution of Calcifications   Grouped/clustered

Clinical History   A 52-year-old woman presents for screening. The patient's mother had breast cancer.

Physical Examination   Normal exam

Radiologic Findings

Mammography

Figure 5–50 Mediolateral (ML) and craniocaudal views. **(A)** Right ML magnification and **(B)** right CC magnification mammograms. There is a cluster of fine pleomorphic calcifications in the upper outer quadrant.

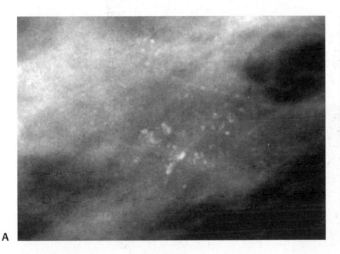
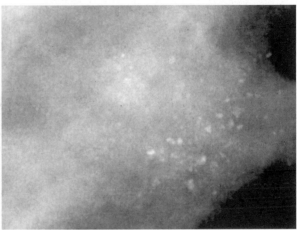

A   B

Management   BI-RADS category 4, suspicious. Biopsy should be considered.

Pathologic Diagnosis

Malignant

DCIS

Pearls and Pitfalls

- These fine pleomorphic calcifications are intermediate suspicion, about a BI-RADS category 4B.

■ Case 5–51

Calcification Morphology   Fine pleomorphic

Distribution of Calcifications   Linear branching

Clinical History   A 54-year-old woman presents for screening.

Physical Examination   Normal exam

Radiologic Findings

Mammography

Figure 5–51 Mediolateral oblique (MLO) and craniocaudal (CC) views. **(A)** Right MLO, **(B)** right CC, **(C)** right MLO magnification, and **(D)** right CC magnification mammograms. There are fine pleomorphic calcifications (*circled*) arranged in a linear branching pattern in the inferior inner breast.

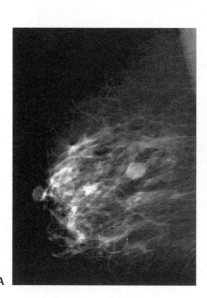 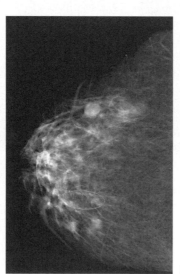 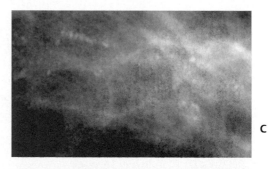 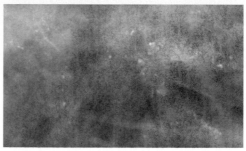

Management   BI-RADS category 5, highly suggestive of malignancy

Pathologic Diagnosis

Malignant

DCIS

Pearls and Pitfalls

- **Figures 5–51A** and **B** demonstrate images that can be created from the screening exam to assist in the later diagnostic additional view workup.

■ Case 5–52

Calcification Morphology   Fine pleomorphic

Distribution of Calcifications   Linear

Clinical History   A 53-year-old woman at screening is found to have new bilateral clustered fine pleomorphic calcifications.

Physical Examination   Bilateral breasts: Normal exam.

Radiologic Findings

Mammography

Figure 5–52 Lateromedial (LM), mediolateral (ML) and craniocaudal (CC) views. **(A)** Right LM magnification mammogram. There is a cluster of fine pleomorphic calcifications in the subareolar region. **(B)** Left CC, **(C)** left ML magnification mammograms, and **(D)** enlargement of **(C)**. There is a cluster of fine pleomorphic calcifications (*arrows*) associated with architectural distortion and irregular mass in the upper outer quadrant.

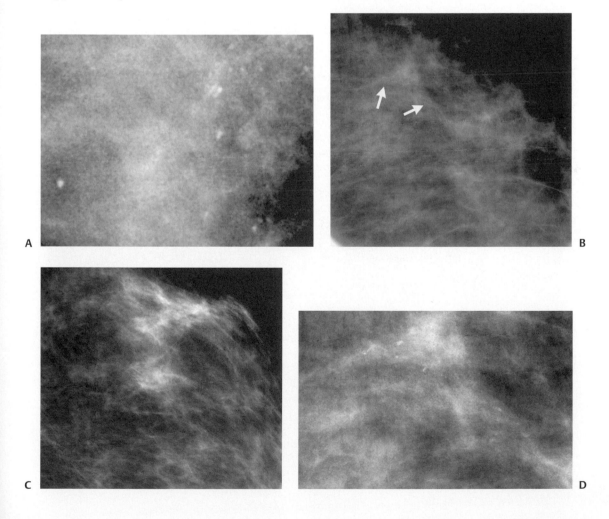

Management   BI-RADS category 5, highly suspicious for malignancy. Appropriate action recommended.

Pathologic Diagnosis

Malignant

Right: DCIS. Left: Invasive ductal carcinoma.

Pearls and Pitfalls

- Simultaneous (synchronous) contralateral malignancy with invasive ductal carcinoma is found in ~3 to 6% of cases.

■ Case 5–53

Calcification Morphology   Fine linear/branching

Distribution of Calcifications   Grouped/clustered

Clinical History   A 55-year-old woman presents for screening.

Physical Examination   Normal exam

Radiologic Findings

Mammography

Figure 5–53 Mediolateral (ML) and craniocaudal (CC) views. **(A)** Right ML magnification and **(B)** right CC magnification mammograms. There is a faint cluster of fine linear branching calcifications (*circled*) near the 6 o'clock position in the right breast.

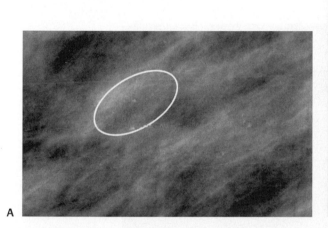
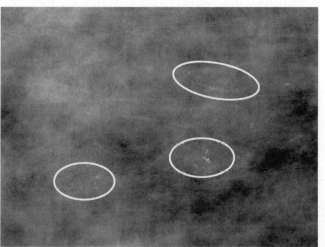

A   B

Management   BI-RADS category 4, suspicious. Biopsy should be considered.

Pathologic Diagnosis

Malignant

DCIS

Comments on Histology   High-grade DCIS with necrosis

Pearls and Pitfalls

- Fine linear branching calcifications are commonly associated with high-grade DCIS with necrosis. These calcifications form within the necrotic center of the duct and extend in a relatively solid path with the tumor. They are also called casting calcifications. This case is a very subtle example of this type of lesion.

■ Case 5–54

Calcification Morphology   Fine linear/branching

Distribution of Calcifications   Segmental

Clinical History   A 41-year-old woman presents for screening.

Physical Examination   After the mammogram was performed, a firm area was identified in the upper outer quadrant.

Radiologic Findings

Mammography

Figure 5–54 Mediolateral oblique (MLO) and craniocaudal (CC) views. **(A)** Right MLO magnification, **(B)** right CC (outer quadrant) magnification, and **(C)** right CC (medial) magnification mammograms. There are fine linear branching calcifications in the right upper outer quadrant **(B)** and at the 3 o'clock position **(C)**. Although the calcifications overlap on the MLO view **(A)**, they are visible as separate areas on the CC view **(B** and **C)**.

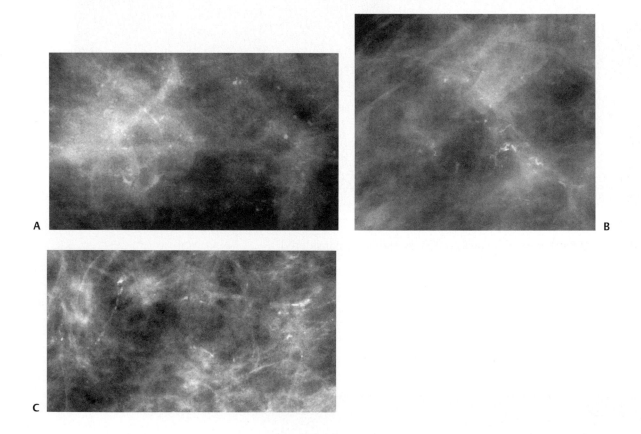

Magnetic Resonance Imaging

Figure 5–54 (D) Three minutes after intravenous gadolinium injection (subtraction series). There are multiple abnormally enhancing areas in the right upper outer quadrant and at the 3 o'clock position.

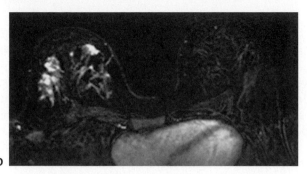

D

Ultrasonography

Figure 5–54 (E) Right breast sonogram. This sonographic mass was one of many suspicious masses that corresponded to the magnetic resonance enhancement.

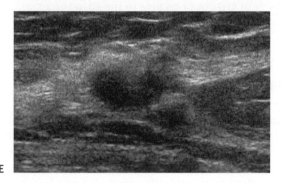

E

Management   BI-RADS category 5, highly suggestive of malignancy

Pathologic Diagnosis

Malignant

Infiltrating ductal carcinoma

Comments on Histology   Stereotaxic biopsy of the calcifications showed high-grade DCIS. Sonographic biopsy of the masses resulted in infiltrating ductal carcinoma. Mastectomy specimen demonstrated 4 cm tumor upper outer quadrant and 2 cm mass at the 3 o'clock position: both infiltrating ductal cancer with extensive intraductal component.

Pearls and Pitfalls

- Multicentricity is generally defined as two neoplasms in different quadrants or at least 5 cm apart. Using this criterion, Lagios and associates found that 28% of 286 cases had multifocal disease.[30]
- Although digital manipulation of screening images commonly provides more information about calcifications, additional magnification views are generally useful, even in highly suspicious cases such as this one. By performing magnification views prior to biopsy, optimal mammographic visualization is available to identify the region of the abnormal calcifications. This information may be used later for needle localization planning or presurgical chemotherapy evaluation.

6 Digital Mammographic Characteristics of Masses

■ Digital Mammographic Technique for Masses

In general, digital mammographic display of breast masses is similar to screen-film.[1] The relatively equivalent visibility is supported by in vitro screen-film and digital mammographic comparison of surgical specimens,[2] as well as prospective clinical evaluation of women with mammographic masses.[3] Multiple studies have addressed the subjective perceptual and diagnostic discrepancies between the two methods. In general, digital mammography produces high-contrast images and reduces the opacity of denser breasts, which increases the confidence of radiologists to exclude masses.[3,4] However these factors as well as slight discrepancies in identification of tumor shape and margin have not produced significant differences in the overall detection of neoplastic masses.[5]

Masses on digital mammography appear similar to those on screen-film images. Although the general workup of digital mammographic masses is similar to screen-film, soft copy viewing allows radiologists to manipulate the screening image more than screen-film. Changing the gray scale window width and level is one of the most useful digital mammographic methods to identify masses. This technique allows masses partially obscured by glandular tissue to be better visualized.[4] This improved conspicuity is important in defining the shape of a mass. Changing the window width and level also improves the identification of any associated suspicious findings, such as architectural distortion, skin thickening, and nipple inversion. Finally, retrospective gray scale manipulation of screening or diagnostic mammographic images can provide useful information to locally stage a biopsy-proven cancer by identifying malignant-appearing satellite masses or calcification clusters.

Digital mammography workstations commonly have computer-aided detection (CAD) software included in their review protocols. CAD appears more sensitive for microcalcifications than for masses. Whereas sensitivities for malignant microcalcifications have been reported as high as ~100%, sensitivities for masses are generally <85%. In general, the CAD sensitivity and specificity increase with larger, more suspicious masses.[6,7]

Magnification of screening images is also useful when characterizing masses. For small masses, magnification may improve the definition of shape and margin. Furthermore, digital enlargement of the mass may provide information that affects further workup. Magnification may demonstrate fat within the mass, which would avoid additional workup. If magnification reveals possible calcifications, the imager may decide to recommend a spot magnification view rather than the nonmagnified spot compression view for the diagnostic workup.

As in the evaluation of calcifications, an important strength of digital mammography is the ability to compare the appearance of masses from earlier digital examinations with the current exam. When masses are small or subtle, digital manipulation is extremely helpful in reproducing similar gray-scale images, which allows more confident assessment of growth or change in the shape of a mass.

■ General Evaluation of Mammographic Mass

As in screen-film, the initial step in a digital mammographic evaluation of a noncalcified lesion is to determine if it is a mass or an asymmetry. A mass has a three-dimensional volume; therefore, it exhibits a consistent shape and density in multiple imaging views or patient positions. Asymmetries tend to be visible only on one view and consist of short concave lines interspersed with tiny lucencies of fat.[8]

After determining that a lesion is a mass, one should determine the shape of the mass. The American College of Radiology's Breast Imaging Reporting and Data System (BI-RADS) defines four shapes: round, oval, lobular, and irregular. However, for purposes of practical assessment, one may divide these shapes into two groups: group 1, low-risk shapes, and group 2, high-risk shapes. Group 1 includes round, oval, and lobular shapes; group 2, irregular shapes. Because of the difference in malignancy risk, each of these groups is treated differently (**Table 6–1**).

When the mass has a group 1 (round, oval, or lobulated) shape, any significant fat within the mass should be identified. Masses with fat, such as lymph nodes, hamartomas, oil cysts, and lipomas, are assessed as BI-RADS category 2, benign, and no further workup is necessary. Even if no fat is present within the mass, further workup may be avoided if there are earlier examination results for comparison, as these masses may be considered benign (BI-RADS category 2) if they have been stable for at least 2 years. Therefore, if earlier exams are readily available, it is important to obtain them.

Table 6–1   Mass Shape Categories

Group 1: Low-Risk Shapes	Group 2: High-Risk Shapes
Round	Irregular
Oval	
Lobular (2–3 lobulations/ 1 cm mass)	

After the initial evaluation, if the mass cannot be determined to be BI-RADS category 2, then the margins of the mass should be evaluated with additional diagnostic mammographic views. Digital spot compression views generally will clarify margins obscured by surrounding parenchyma. Magnification spot compression views will also improve the characterization of margins when masses are extremely tiny.[9,10]

If the group 1 mass does not contain fat, then the mass should be sonographically examined to determine if it is cystic or solid. Group 1 masses that have circumscribed, microlobulated, obscured, or indistinct margins should all be sonographically examined. If the mass is cystic, then the lesion should be assessed BI-RADS category 2, benign.

If the mass is sonographically occult or solid, then it should be characterized on the basis of the most suspicious mammographic or sonographic findings. A detailed review of the sonographic assessment of solid masses is beyond the scope of this discussion. However, in general, if the mass is nonpalpable, has a group 1 shape with a completely circumscribed margin, and has no other associated suspicious mammographic or sonographic findings, then it is assessed as BI-RADS category 3, probably benign, and a short-interval follow-up is suggested (**Table 6–2**). Previous screen-film studies have shown that ~2 to 3% of mixed screening and diagnostic patients have circumscribed group 1 masses, and between 0.4 and 1.4% of well-circumscribed masses are malignant.[11–15]

Mammographic group 1 masses that are sonographically occult and are not circumscribed should be biopsied. Suspicious margin characteristics, including microlobulated, obscured, indistinct, and spiculated, should be biopsied.[16]

If the margins of the mammographic group 1 mass are spiculated, and the mass is associated with other highly

Table 6–2   BI-RADS Assessments for Mammographic Masses

BI-RADS Assessment	Definition	Examples of Mammographic Mass Findings
Category 1	Negative	No mass present; "pseudomass" due to overlap of normal fibroglandular tissue
Category 2	Benign finding	Round, oval, gently lobulated circumscribed mass stable for 2 years or smaller than previous exams
		Fat containing round, oval, gently lobulated circumscribed masses
		Known scar (irregular mass) stable or smaller
		Benign sonographic mass (cyst, lymph node)
Category 3	Probably benign finding; initial short-term interval follow-up suggested	New round, oval, or gently lobulated well-circumscribed mass (solid or not sonographically visible; not palpable); no associated suspicious mammographic finding (see Category 5). No associated suspicious sonographic findings: shadowing, spiculations, angular margins, echogenic halo, microlobulations, nonparallel orientation, duct extension, branch pattern, or calcification[15]
Category 4	Suspicious abnormality—biopsy should be considered	
Category 4A		Growing round, oval, lobular solid, or sonographically occult mass with circumscribed or circumscribed with partially obscured margins
Category 4B		Round, oval, lobular solid, or sonographically occult mass with indistinct or microlobulated margins
Category 4C		Irregular mass with ill-defined margins
Category 5	Highly suspicious of malignancy	Irregular high-density mass with spiculated margin (other associated findings: architectural distortion, skin thickening, nipple inversion, trabecular thickening, skin retraction, or malignant microcalcifications)

BI-RADS, Breast Imaging Reporting and Data System.

suspicious findings (BI-RADS category 5), then the lesion should be assessed as highly suggestive of malignancy, and appropriate action should be taken. In these cases, sonography may be performed to plan biopsy guidance.

Group 2 (irregular) masses are treated differently from group 1 masses. Although spot compression views are useful in clarifying the size and location of these masses, unlike group 1 masses, defining the margin will not avoid biopsy. If a group 2 mass is new or growing, then this lesion is assessed at least BI-RADS category 4, suspicious. If the irregular mass is clearly identified mammographically, then sonographically the mass will generally also appear suspicious. Sonography may be used primarily to plan biopsy. Irregular masses are generally more suspicious than circumscribed ones, and those irregular masses that are spiculated and associated with other highly suspicious findings tend to form BI-RADS category 5, highly suggestive of malignancy (**Table 6–2**).

Differentiating BI-RADS category 4 (particularly category 4C) from category 5 masses is subjective and based on experience and constant retrospective review correlating assessment with histology data. Therefore, depending on the patient population, the criteria for categories 4A, 4B, 4C, and 5 will differ between institutions. **Table 6–2** is a general guide outlining the most common characteristics of masses in each assessment category. The general order of these characteristics is inferred from multiple retrospective studies. However, other than BI-RADS category 2 and 3 characteristics, studies have not clearly defined any specific single finding or combination of findings that consistently will translate to the generally accepted BI-RADS risks for category 4A (low suspicion: 3–33%), category 4B (intermediate suspicion: 34–64%), category 4C (moderate suspicion: 65–94%), and category 5 (high suspicion: ≥95%). Multiple studies have noted that spiculated or highly irregular shapes tend to have the highest association with malignancy.[17–19] Although high density is commonly cited as an important characteristic of a mammographic mass, this finding is poorly predictive of malignancy.[20]

One irregular mass that is treated differently from the rest is the postsurgical or traumatic scar.[21] When performing screening mammography, the radiologist should be informed of any previous surgical or invasive breast procedures. If one is not sure that the irregular mass is a scar, then comparison with previous examinations is extremely important. Comparing the appearance of scars between digital mammo-grams and screen-film mammograms is a challenge because there is often a subtle difference in brightness and contrast, which may cause the scar to appear more conspicuous on digital mammography. If the scar has been stable for at least 2 years or has decreased in size, then the irregular mass may be assessed as category 2, benign. If the irregular mass is new or getting larger, then the mass should be assessed as category 4, suspicious, and biopsy is recommended. Sonography is useful in guiding biopsy in these lesions.

Once a mammographic mass has been identified, many radiologists sonographically examine the mass to improve characterization. Sonography characterization of masses is so automatic that many radiologists proceed directly to ultrasound without evaluation of the mammographic margins of a mass. However, although this method may save time, one should be aware of the pitfalls. The most serious error that may result from inadequate mammographic evaluation of the margins of a mass is misassessment of the lesion. For example, a radiologist may send a patient with a group 1 circumscribed mass on a screening exam directly to ultrasound. In this case, there may be subtle mammographic architectural distortion or spiculation that is only evident on additional mammographic views. When these diagnostic mammographic images are not performed, these suspicious findings may be missed. Furthermore, these abnormalities may not be visible sonographically, causing the mass to be misassessed as category 3, probably benign. This situation poses serious consequences for patients with small high-grade infiltrating ductal cancers that sometimes appear as sonographically cystic or circumscribed solid masses. Obviously, a mass with mammographic spiculated margins or architectural distortion should be assessed as category 4, suspicious, or category 5, highly suggestive of malignancy, even if the mass has sonographically well-defined margins.

Skipping the mammographic characterization of a mass may lead to another potential problem. If the mammographic mass is not identified sonographically, then the assessment should be based on the mammographic appearance of the mass. For a group 1 circumscribed mass, digital manipulation of screening images may clarify the mass's shape. However, these maneuvers generally do not replace careful diagnostic imaging to evaluate the margins of the mass, so the radiologist may need to send the patient for additional mammographic views if the sonographic exam is negative.

References

1. Fischer U, Hermann KP, Baum F. Digital mammography: current state and future aspects. Eur Radiol 2006;16:38–44
2. Kuzmiak CM, Millnamow GA, Qaqish B, Pisano ED, Cole EB, Brown ME. Comparison of full-field digital mammography to screen-film mammography with respect to diagnostic accuracy of lesion characterization in breast tissue biopsy specimens. Acad Radiol 2002;9:1378–1382
3. Fischmann A, Siegmann KC, Wersebe A, Claussen CD, Muller-Schimpfle M. Comparison of full-field digital mammography and film-screen mammography: image quality and lesion detection. Br J Radiol 2005;78:312–315
4. Obenauer S, Luftner-Nagel S, Von Heyden D, Munzel U, Baum F, Grabbe E. Screen film vs full-field digital mammography: image quality, detectability and characterization of lesions. Eur Radiol 2002;12:1697–1702
5. Lewin JM, D'Orsi CJ, Hendrick RE, et al. Clinical comparison of full-field digital mammography and screen-film mammography for detection of breast cancer. Am J Roentgenol 2002;179:671–677

6. Obenauer S, Sohns C, Werner C, Grabbe E. Computer-aided detection in full-field digital mammography: detection in dependence of the BI-RADS categories. Breast J 2006;12:16–19

7. Brem RF, Hoffmeister JW, Zisman G, DeSimio MP, Rogers SK. A computer-aided detection system for the evaluation of breast cancer by mammographic appearance and lesion size. Am J Roentgenol 2005;184:893–896

8. Sickles EA. Breast masses: mammographic evaluation. Radiology 1989;173:297–303

9. Berkowitz JE, Gatewood OMB, Gayler BW. Equivocal mammographic findings: evaluation with spot compression. Radiology 1989;171:369–371

10. Sickles EA. Combining spot-compression and other special views to maximize mammographic information [letter]. Radiology 1989;173:571

11. Varas X, Leborgne F, Leborgne JH. Nonpalpable, probably benign lesions: role of follow-up mammography. Radiology 1992;184:409–414

12. Sickles EA. Nonpalpable, circumscribed, noncalcified solid breast masses: likelihood of malignancy based on lesion size and age of patient. Radiology 1994;192:439–442

13. Varas X, Leborgne JH, Leborgne F, Mezzera J, Jaumandreu S, Leborgne F. Revisiting the mammographic follow-up of BI-RADS category 3 lesions. Am J Roentgenol 2002;179: 691–695

14. Vizcaino I, Gadea L, Andreo L, et al. Short-term follow-up results in 795 nonpalpable probably benign lesions detected at screening mammography. Radiology 2001;219:475–483

15. Stavros AT. Ultrasound of solid breast nodules: distinguishing benign from malignant. In: Breast Ultrasound. Philadelphia: Lippincott Williams & Wilkins; 2004:445–527

16. Tot T, Tabar L, Dean PB. Fine-needle aspiration or core biopsy: a preoperative diagnostic algorithm. In: Practical Breast Pathology. New York: Thieme; 2002:99–123

17. Hall FM, Storella JM, Silverstone DZ, Wyshak G. Nonpalpable breast lesions: recommendations for biopsy based on suspicion of carcinoma at mammography. Radiology 1988;167: 353–358

18. Liberman L, Abramson AF, Squires FB, Glassman JR, Morris EA, Dershaw DD. The breast imaging reporting and data system: positive predictive value of mammographic features and final assessment categories. Am J Roentgenol 1998;171:35–40

19. Ciatto S, Cataliotti L, Distante V. Nonpalpable lesions detected with mammography: review of 512 consecutive cases. Radiology 1987;165:99–102

20. Jackson VP, Dines KA, Bassett LW, Gold RH, Reynolds HE. Diagnostic importance of the radiographic density of noncalcified breast masses: analysis of 91 lesions. Am J Roentgenol 1991;157: 25–28

21. Sickles EA, Herzog KA. Intramammary scar tissue: a mimic of the mammographic appearance of carcinoma. Am J Roentgenol 1980;135:349–352

22. Sickles EA. Practical solutions to common mammographic problems: tailoring the examination. Am J Roentgenol 1988;151: 31–39

■ Case 6–1

Characteristics of Masses   Circumscribed masses

Clinical History   A 45-year-old woman presents for screening.

Physical Examination   Normal exam

Radiologic Findings

Mammography

Figure 6–1 Mediolateral oblique (MLO) and craniocaudal (CC) views. **(A)** Right MLO and **(B)** right CC mammograms. There is an oval circumscribed mass (*arrow*) at the 9 o'clock position. This mass has been stable for more than 3 years. The mass has a mixture of fat and fibroglandular density. The small central circumscribed mass on the CC view is a cyst, identified by an earlier sonographic exam.

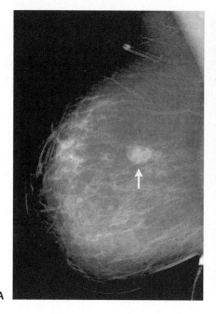
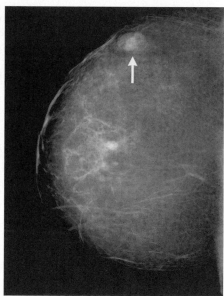

A   B

Management   BI-RADS category 2, benign finding

Pathologic Diagnosis

Benign

Hamartoma

Pearls and Pitfalls

- Hamartomas are benign tumors that consist of mature cells that normally occur in the breast. Mammographically, their appearance varies depending on the amount of fat within the mass. They have been described as having a "cut sausage" or "breast within the breast" appearance, because the fibroglandular tissues tend to form clumps surrounded by fat. Digital manipulation of the image is useful in this lesion to better identify the fatty regions and the tumor's pseudocapsule.

■ Case 6–2

Characteristics of Masses   Circumscribed masses

Clinical History   A 42-year-old woman presents for screening.

Physical Examination   Normal exam

Radiologic Findings

Mammography

Figure 6–2 Mediolateral oblique (MLO) and craniocaudal (CC) views. **(A)** Right MLO and **(B)** right CC mammograms. In the right upper breast on the MLO view (*arrow*), there is an oval circumscribed mass.

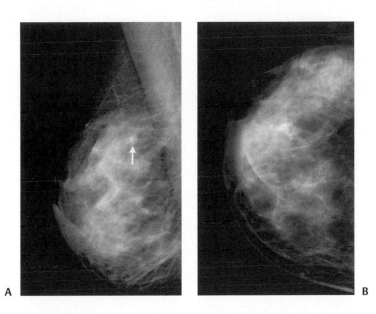

A   B

Ultrasonography

Figure 6–2 (C) Right breast sonogram and **(D)** right breast color Doppler sonogram. The mammographic oval mass corresponds to a benign-appearing lymph node. The color Doppler image confirms the benign internal architecture of the node. The cortex is uniform, and the hilum is centrally located. Lymph node (N), fat (F) normal glandular tissue (G).

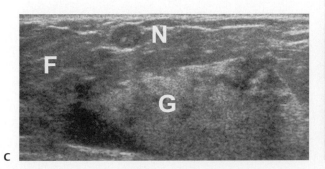

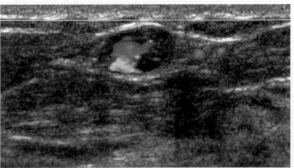

C   D

Management   BI-RADS category 2, benign finding

Pathologic Diagnosis

Benign

Lymph node

Pearls and Pitfalls

- This case demonstrates cross-correlation between digital mammographic anatomy and ultrasound. **Figure 6–2A** demonstrates that the node is surrounded by fat and separated from dense glandular tissue, so it appears well circumscribed on the mammographic MLO view.

■ Case 6–3

Characteristics of Masses   Circumscribed masses

Clinical History   A 71-year-old woman presents with a palpable right breast lump. She cannot remember any trauma.

Physical Examination   Right breast: Lump at the 4 o'clock position.

Radiologic Findings

Mammography

Figure 6–3 Mediolateral oblique (MLO) and craniocaudal (CC) views. **(A)** Right MLO, **(B)** right CC, **(C)** right MLO spot compression, and **(D)** right CC spot compression. There is a circumscribed fat density mass at the 4 o'clock position.

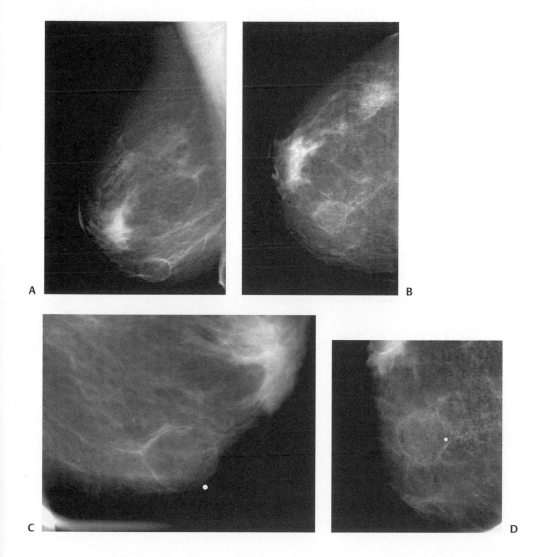

Ultrasonography

Figure 6–3 (E) Right breast sonogram. The palpable mammographic mass is a cystic mass with a thick wall. This complex cyst is consistent with an oil cyst.

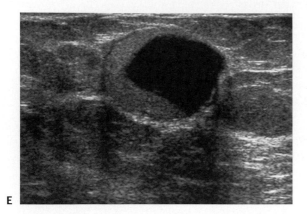

E

Management   BI-RADS category 2, benign finding

Pathologic Diagnosis

Benign

Oil cyst

Pearls and Pitfalls

- Normally, no sonographic exam would be necessary to confirm an oil cyst. In this case, the sonographic exam was performed to confirm that the palpable lump directly corresponded to the oil cyst. Note that sonographically oil cysts present as complex cysts. They should not be considered suspicious if their mammographic appearance is pathognomonic for oil cysts.

■ Case 6–4

Characteristics of Masses   Circumscribed masses

Clinical History   A 65-year-old woman presents for screening.

Physical Examination   Right chest: Pacemaker palpated.

Radiologic Findings

Mammography

Figure 6–4 Mediolateral (ML) and craniocaudal (CC) views. **(A)** Right ML and **(B)** right CC mammograms. There is a radiopaque foreign body consistent with a pacemaker overlying the breast.

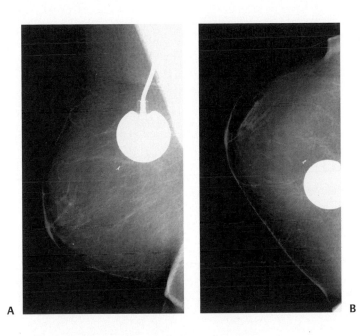

A   B

Management   BI-RADS category 1, negative

Pathologic Diagnosis

Benign

Foreign body: Pacemaker

Pearls and Pitfalls

- Foreign bodies are generally easily identified by their radiographic metallic density. Bullets or bullet fragments, needles, and wires have been reported mammographically.

■ Case 6–5

Characteristics of Masses   Circumscribed masses

History   A 48-year-old woman presents for screening.

Physical Examination   Normal exam

Radiologic Findings

Mammography

Figure 6–5 Mediolateral oblique (MLO) and craniocaudal (CC) views. **(A)** Right MLO and **(B)** right CC mammograms. There is an oval circumscribed mass in the upper outer quadrant. A lucent halo encircles the medial anterior margin.

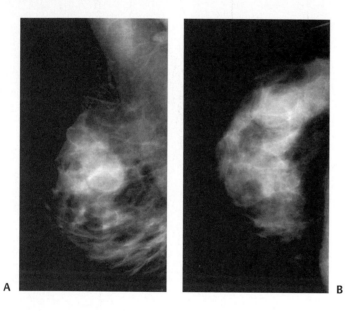

Ultrasonography

Figure 6–5 **(C)** Right breast sonogram. The mammographic mass corresponds to a simple cyst.

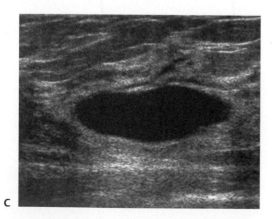

Management   BI-RADS category 2, benign finding

Pathologic Diagnosis

Benign

Cyst

Pearls and Pitfalls

- Cysts are the most common type of mass in women between the ages of 40 and 50 years. Researchers have estimated that 7 to 10% of all women have cysts. Mammographically, cysts are well-circumscribed, low- or equal-density masses that are round, oval, or lobular. The benignity of these lesions is further suggested by the halo sign.

■ Case 6–6

Characteristics of Masses   Circumscribed masses

Clinical History   A 54-year-old woman presents with a new right breast lump at the 11 o'clock position.

Physical Examination   Right breast: About 1 cm lump at the 11 o'clock position.

Radiologic Findings

Mammography

Figure 6–6 Mediolateral oblique (MLO) and craniocaudal (CC) views. **(A)** Right MLO and **(B)** right CC mammograms. There is an oval well-circumscribed mass at the 11 o'clock position (*arrows*).

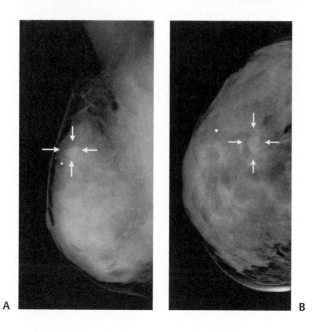

A   B

Ultrasonography

Figure 6–6 (C) Right breast sonogram. The palpable lump corresponds to a cyst. The sonogram is performed with a standoff pad because the cyst is extremely superficial. The palpable nature of the cyst is emphasized, as the cyst protrudes outside the normal contour of the breast. Although there is one thin septation, the cyst is otherwise simple and is therefore benign.

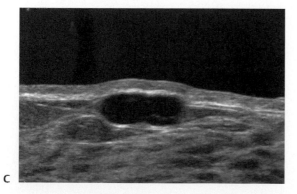

C

Management   BI-RADS category 2, benign finding

Pathologic Diagnosis

Benign

Cyst

Pearls and Pitfalls

- Because mammographic cysts cannot be differentiated from other solid masses, these circumscribed masses are best characterized sonographically. Sonography has been found to be between 96 and 100% accurate in identifying cysts.

■ Case 6–7

Characteristics of Masses   Circumscribed masses

Clinical History   New asymmetric density is seen in the left craniocaudal view only.

Physical Examination   Normal exam

Radiologic Findings

Mammography

Figure 6–7   Mediolateral oblique (MLO) and craniocaudal (CC) views. **(A)** Left CC and **(B)** left MLO mammograms. In the medial aspect of the CC view, there is an oval asymmetry within some asymmetric breast tissue. Although the asymmetric breast tissue is stable, the oval asymmetry is new since the previous exam. **(C)** Left CC (same image as **(A)**. **(D)** Left 20-degree MLO. **(E)** Left 40-degree MLO (same image as **(B)**. The oval asymmetry is medial on the CC view (*arrow*), but the shallow oblique view shows that the oval asymmetry "moves" toward the upper breast (*arrow*). Therefore, in retrospect, the asymmetry can be localized on the original MLO view; this asymmetry represents an oval circumscribed mass in the inner upper quadrant (*arrow*).

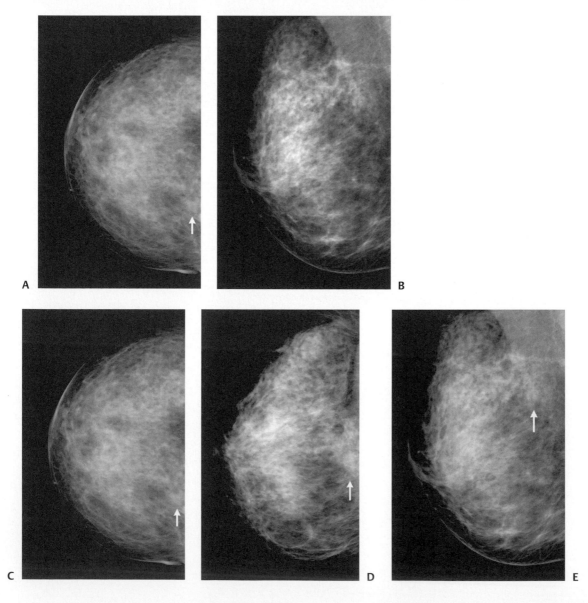

A   B

C   D   E

Ultrasonography

Figure 6–7 (F) Left breast sonogram. Once the circumscribed mass was localized mammographically, it was sonographically examined and found to be a simple cyst.

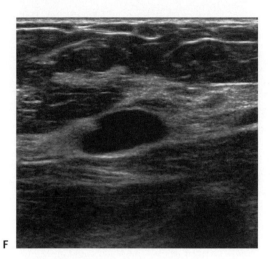

F

Management　　BI-RADS category 2, benign finding

Pathologic Diagnosis

Benign

Cyst

Pearls and Pitfalls

- When an asymmetry cannot be identified in more than one view, an operator-independent method to localize a mass is performed. This technique, as described by Sickles, involves shallow oblique views. If the mass is visible only in the CC view, then 10- and 20-degree MLO views are done. These views are positioned horizontally on the workstation monitors in this order: CC, 10-degree MLO, 20-degree MLO, and original MLO. The position of each of these images must be adjusted so that the nipples form a horizontal line. The lesion is first localized on the CC view and then identified on the shallow oblique views. Notice the relative shift in position of the lesion compared to the nipple with each oblique view. The lesion's shifting position will follow one of three patterns: stay in the retroareolar plane or move superior or inferior to the nipple line. If the lesion moves superiorly, it will probably be in the outer breast in the original MLO view. If it moves inferiorly, it will be in the medial breast on the MLO. If it is retroareolar, it will be close to central on the original MLO view.[22] (See Chapter 7, pp. 149–151.)

■ Case 6–8

Characteristics of Masses   Circumscribed masses

Clinical History   A 52-year-old woman presents for screening.

Physical Examination   Normal exam

Radiologic Findings

Mammography

Figure 6–8 Mediolateral oblique (MLO) and craniocaudal (CC) views. **(A)** Left MLO and **(B)** left CC mammograms. At the 3 o'clock position, there is a partially obscured, oval mass (*circled*), which is new since the patient's previous exam.

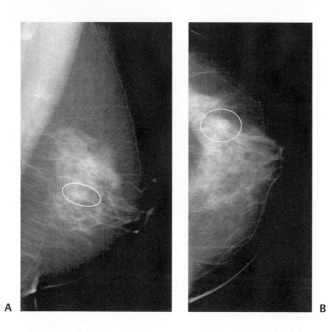

A   B

Ultrasonography

Figure 6–8 (C) Left breast sonogram. The mammographic mass corresponds to an oval mass with slightly irregular borders. There are diffuse low-level internal echoes and no increased through transmission. This mass was interpreted as being solid. **(D)** With the first biopsy needle pass, the hypoechoic mass in **(C)** collapsed. A sonographic reexamination of the breast 6 months later demonstrated no evidence of the mass.

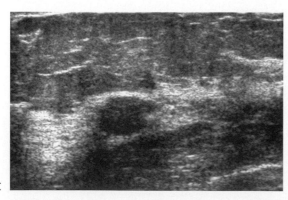

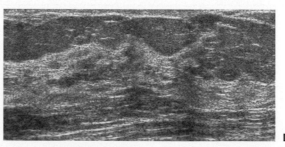

C   D

Management   BI-RADS category 4, suspicious. Biopsy should be considered.

Pathologic Diagnosis

Benign

Cyst

Pearls and Pitfalls

- A pitfall of sonographically examining mammographic circumscribed masses is that benign cysts may look like solid masses. Furthermore, if the margins are mildly irregular, they should be assessed as suspicious—usually BI-RADS category 4A.

■ Case 6–9

Characteristics of Masses   Circumscribed masses

Clinical History   A 45-year-old woman presents with a new right mammo-graphic mass.

Physical Examination   Normal exam

Radiologic Findings

Mammography

Figure 6–9 Mediolateral oblique (MLO) and craniocaudal (CC) views. **(A)** Right MLO and **(B)** right CC mammograms. There is an oval circumscribed mass at the 9 o'clock position. **(C)** Right MLO and **(D)** right CC mammograms. These mammograms are the same views as **(A)** and **(B)**, but they have been electronically marked and saved in the patient's digital file.

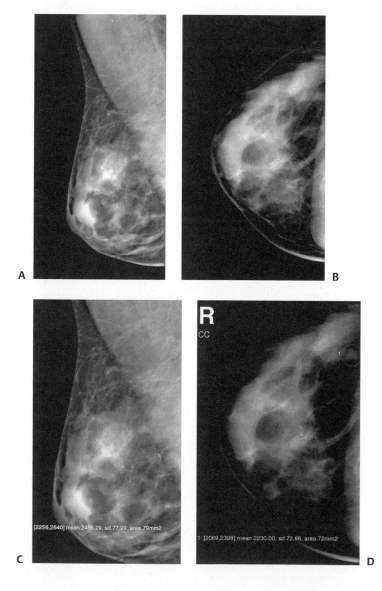

Ultrasonography

Figure 6–9 (E) Right breast sonogram. The mammographic mass corresponds to a simple cyst with one thin septation.

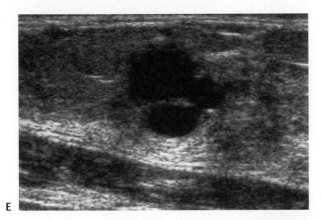

E

Management   BI-RADS category 2, benign finding

Pathologic Diagnosis

Benign

Cyst

Pearls and Pitfalls

- Electronically marked images are useful to guide later workup of a patient. These images created at the time of the screening may either be saved in the patient's permanent file or printed and not electronically stored.
- Sonographically, simple cysts with a thin septation are benign. There should not be any color Doppler signal within the septation, and there should not be any wall thickening, asymmetric thickening of the septation, or associated soft tissue masses.

■ Case 6–10

Characteristics of Masses Circumscribed masses

Clinical History A 54-year-old woman presents for screening.

Physical Examination Normal exam

Radiologic Findings

Mammography

Figure 6–10 Mediolateral oblique (MLO) and craniocaudal (CC) views. **(A)** Left spot compression MLO and **(B)** left spot compression CC mammograms. At the 5 o'clock position, there is an oval circumscribed mass.

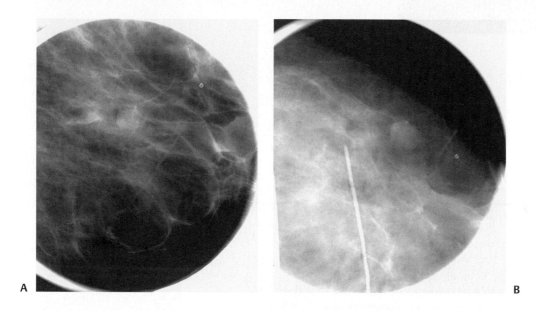

A   B

Ultrasonography

Figure 6–10 (C) Left breast sonogram. The mammographic mass corresponds to a cyst with a thick septation. **(D)** Left breast color Doppler sonogram. There is an abnormal color Doppler signal within the thick cystic septation.

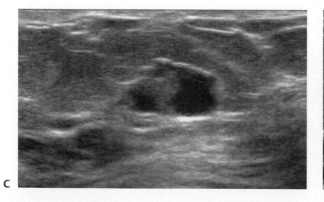
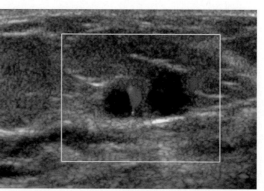

C   D

Management   BI-RADS category 4, suspicious. Biopsy should be considered.

Pathologic Diagnosis

Benign

Apocrine metaplasia

Comments on Histology   The initial ultrasound-guided biopsy produced an incidental focus of atypical ductal hyperplasia (ADH), so the mass was excised. There was no additional ADH, only cyst formation and apocrine metaplasia

---

Pearls and Pitfalls

- The final assessment of this lesion was based on the sonographic findings. Whenever a cystic mass has a thick septation and/or color Doppler signal within the septation, the lesion should be assessed as suspicious—usually BI-RADS category 4A.

■ Case 6–11

Characteristics of Masses   Circumscribed masses

Clinical History   A 48-year-old presents with a palpable left breast lump.

Physical Examination   Left breast: Lump at the 2 o'clock position.

Radiologic Findings

Mammography

Figure 6–11 Mediolateral oblique (MLO) and craniocaudal (CC) views. **(A)** Left MLO and **(B)** left CC mammograms. There is an oval circumscribed mass at the 2 o'clock position that corresponds to the palpable mass identified by the radiographic skin marker.

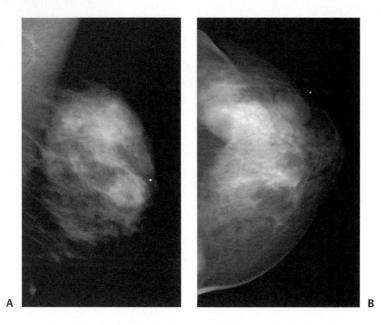

A   B

Ultrasonography

Figure 6–11 (C) Left breast sonogram. The mammographic and palpable mass corresponds to an oval circumscribed solid mass. Although the sonographic findings of this mass are probably benign, this mass was assessed as suspicious because it had exhibited rapid growth since the patient's previous screening exam and was now palpable.

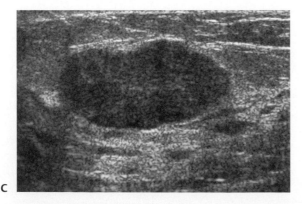

C

Management   BI-RADS category 4, suspicious. Biopsy should be considered.

Pathologic Diagnosis

Benign

Fibroadenoma

Pearls and Pitfalls

- Fibroadenomas reach a maximal incidence in women ages 20 to 30 and generally involute after menopause. If a solid circumscribed mass increases in size in a post-menopausal woman, the lesion should be considered suspicious.

■ Case 6–12

Characteristics of Masses   Circumscribed masses

Clinical History   A 39-year-old woman presents with a palpable left breast lump.

Physical Examination   Left breast: Palpable lump at the 9 o'clock position.

Radiologic Findings

Mammography

Figure 6–12   Mediolateral oblique (MLO) and craniocaudal (CC) views. **(A)** Left MLO, **(B)** left CC, and **(C)** left spot compression MLO mammograms. At the 9 o'clock position, there is an oval circumscribed mass (*arrows*) with a lucent halo.

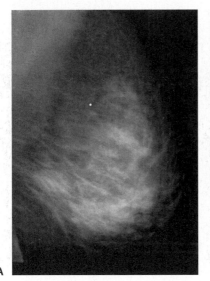
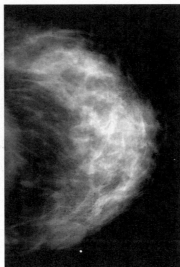
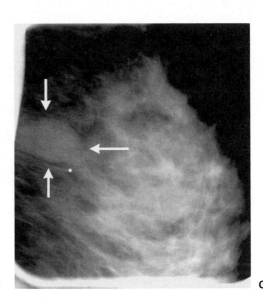

Ultrasonography

Figure 6–12 (D) Left breast radial and **(E)** left breast antiradial sonogram. The mammographic mass and the palpable mass correspond to a solid mass that is oval in the radial orientation but irregular in the antiradial plane.

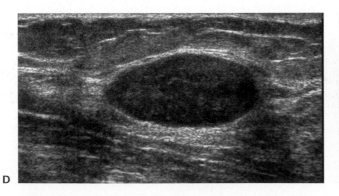
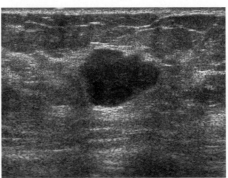

Management   BI-RADS category 4, suspicious. Biopsy should be considered.

Pathologic Diagnosis

Benign

Fibroadenoma

Pearls and Pitfalls

- Mammographically, fibroadenomas appear similar to cysts: they are well-circumscribed round, oval, or lobulated, equal- or low-density masses. Fibroadenomas, like cysts, may also have lucent halos (see Case 6–5).

■ Case 6–13

Characteristics of Masses   Circumscribed masses

Clinical History   A 58-year-old woman presents with a left breast lump.

Physical Examination   Left breast: Lump at the 9 o'clock position.

Radiologic Findings

Mammography

Figure 6–13 Mediolateral oblique (MLO) and craniocaudal (CC) views. **(A)** Left MLO, **(B)** left CC, **(C)** left MLO spot compression, and **(D)** left CC spot compression mammograms. Near the 9 o'clock position, there is an oval circumscribed mass. The CC spot compression **(D)** demonstrates this mass protruding from the breast.

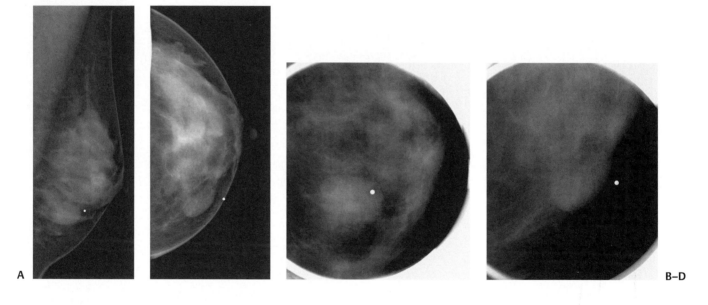

Ultrasonography

Figure 6–13 **(E)** Left breast radial sonogram and **(F)** left breast antiradial sonogram. The palpable mammographic mass corresponds to an oval isoechoic mass. Although most of the margin is well defined, the mass exhibits mild irregularity of the margin, particularly in the antiradial orientation.

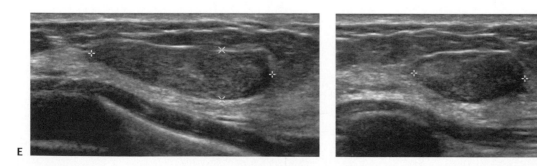

Management   BI-RADS category 4, suspicious. Biopsy should be considered.

Pathologic Diagnosis

Benign

Pseudoangiomatous stromal hyperplasia (PASH)

Pearls and Pitfalls

- Clinically, PASH presents as a palpable mass in 50% of cases. It generally appears as a circumscribed mammographic and sonographic mass.

■ Case 6–14

Characteristics of Masses   Circumscribed masses

Clinical History   A 66-year-old woman has a right breast lump.

Physical Examination   Right breast: Lump at about the 9 o'clock position.

Radiologic Findings

Mammography

Figure 6–14 Mediolateral oblique (MLO) and craniocaudal (CC) views. **(A)** Right MLO and **(B)** right CC mammograms. There is an oval mass at the 9 o'clock position. The margins are partially ill defined.

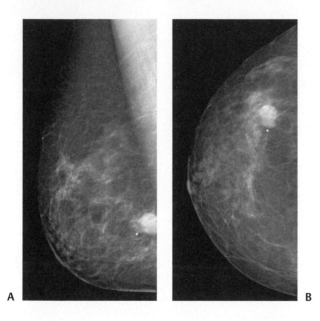

A   B

Ultrasonography

Figure 6–14 (C) Right breast sonogram. The palpable lump and the mammographic mass correspond to a hypoechoic lobulated mass with mildly irregular and ill-defined margins.

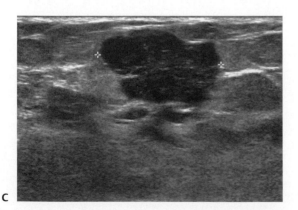

C

Management   BI-RADS category 4, suspicious. Biopsy should be considered.

Pathologic Diagnosis

Malignant

Invasive ductal carcinoma

Pearls and Pitfalls

- Invasive ductal carcinoma is the most common malignancy that presents as an oval, round, or lobulated mass. Other malignancies that present in this manner include medullary cancer, mucinous cancer, papillary cancer, metastases, phyllode tumor, and intracystic cancer.

■ Case 6–15

Characteristics of Masses   Circumscribed masses

History   A 53-year-old woman presents with left breast and axillary tenderness that has lasted for 3 months.

Physical Examination   Left breast: Palpable mass in upper outer quadrant; also palpable axillary adenopathy.

Radiologic Findings

Mammography

Figure 6–15 Mediolateral oblique (MLO) and craniocaudal (CC) views. **(A)** Left MLO, **(B)** left CC, and **(C)** left axillary MLO spot compression mammograms. There is an ill-defined oval mass in the upper outer quadrant of the left breast associated with axillary adenopathy.

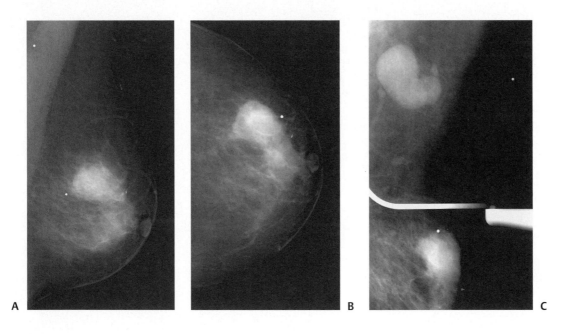

A   B   C

Ultrasonography

Figure 6–15 (D) Left breast sonogram. The mammographic breast mass corresponds to a solid ill-defined mass with irregular borders. **(E)** Left axillary sonogram. The mammographically enlarged lymph node corresponds to a large lobulated lymph node with irregularly thickened cortex.

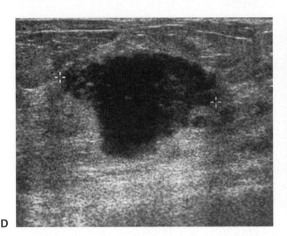
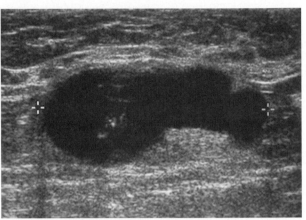

D   E

Magnetic Resonance Imaging

Figure 6–15 (F) Bilateral breast MRI (subtraction series: 2 minutes after injection of contrast). The left mammographic mass corresponds to an early enhancing oval mass. The mammographically and sonographically abnormal lymph node also exhibited malignant enhancement.

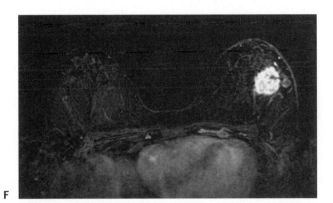

F

Management   BI-RADS category 5, highly suspicious for malignancy. Biopsy should be considered.

Pathologic Diagnosis

Malignant

Invasive ductal carcinoma

Comments on Histology   Enlarged lymph node also exhibited metastatic disease.

Pearls and Pitfalls

- Lymph nodes usually are circumscribed oval masses with a central fatty hilum. As they enlarge, they become lobular and lose their normal internal fatty hilum. Some malignant nodes exhibit malignant calcifications.

■ Case 6–16

Characteristics of Masses   Circumscribed masses

Clinical History   A 57-year-old woman presents for screening and is found to have a new left mass. She has a breast sonogram in which the mammographic mass is interpreted as a cyst. She returns 5 months later with a palpable left breast lump and has another breast sonogram.

Physical Examination   Left breast: At second visit, the patient has a lump at the 2 o'clock position.

Radiologic Findings

Mammography

Figure 6–16 Mediolateral oblique (MLO) and craniocaudal (CC) views. **(A)** Left MLO and **(B)** left CC mammograms. There is an oval mass with ill-defined margins in the upper outer quadrant. Breast sonogram of this mass was interpreted as a cyst. **(C)** Left MLO and **(D)** left CC mammograms. The patient returns 5 months later with a palpable mass that corresponds to an oval high-density mass at the 2 o'clock position. Left breast sonogram was repeated.

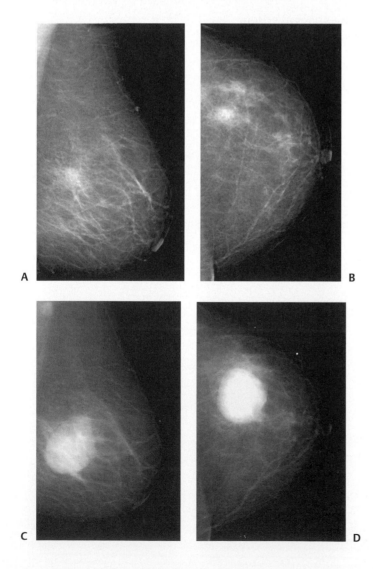

A   B

C   D

Ultrasonography

Figure 6–16 **(E)** Left breast sonogram. Patient's initial sonogram demonstrated an anechoic oval mass that corresponded to the mammographic mass. This mass was interpreted as a cyst. **(F,G)** Left breast sonograms performed 5 months after **(E)**. The anechoic mass has increased in size. Some parts of the mass are still anechoic and have increased sound transmission **(F)**. However, most of the mass appears to have coarse thick septations and thickened irregular walls **(G)**.

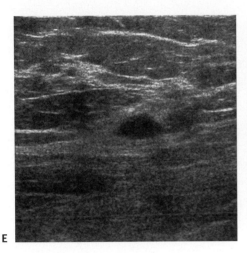

E

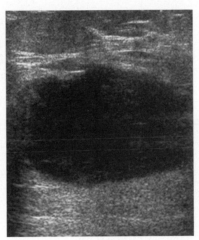

F

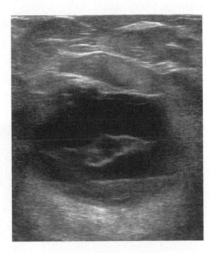

G

Management   BI-RADS category 4, suspicious. Biopsy should be considered.

Pathologic Diagnosis

Malignant

Metaplastic carcinoma

Pearls and Pitfalls

- The increased sound transmission associated with the oval circumscribed appearance led to the erroneous sonographic diagnosis of a simple cyst. Invasive malignancies that produce increased sound transmission include high-grade invasive ductal carcinoma, colloid carcinoma, medullary carcinoma, papillary carcinoma, and metaplastic carcinoma. However, these malignancies usually are associated with irregular shapes and ill-defined margins.
- Metaplastic carcinoma consists of heterogeneous tumors that contain epithelial or mesenchymal components in addition to the mammary adenocarcinoma.

■ Case 6–17

Characteristics of Masses   Circumscribed masses

Clinical History   A 91-year-old woman presents with a palpable left breast lump.

Physical Examination   Left breast: Lump near the 9 o'clock position.

Radiologic Findings

Mammography

Figure 6–17 Mediolateral oblique (MLO) and craniocaudal (CC) views. **(A)** Left MLO and **(B)** left CC mammograms. Near the 9 o'clock position there is a high density oval mass.

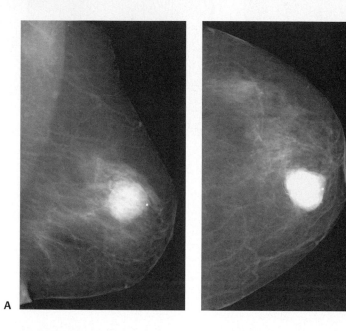

A   B

Ultrasonography

Figure 6–17 **(C)** Left breast sonogram. The palpable mammographic mass corresponds to a solid hypoechoic mass with mildly irregular margins.

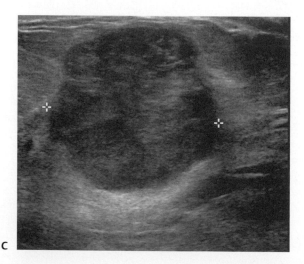

C

Management   BI-RADS category 4, suspicious. Biopsy should be considered.

Pathologic Diagnosis

Malignant

Invasive papillary carcinoma

Pearls and Pitfalls

- Central papillary carcinoma tends to be solitary, well-defined, oval, or lobulated masses.
- Presenting symptoms include palpable lump (90%), nipple discharge (25%), and nipple distortion/retraction (28%).

■ Case 6–18

Characteristics of Masses   Circumscribed masses

Clinical History   A 66-year-old woman presents for screening; she has a possible change in a right mammographic breast mass.

Physical Examination   Normal exam

Radiologic Findings

Mammography

Figure 6–18 Mediolateral oblique (MLO) and craniocaudal (CC) views. **(A)** Right MLO and **(B)** right CC mammograms performed 2 years prior to the current exam. In the 7 o'clock position, there is a high-density oval mass (*arrow*). **(C)** Right MLO and **(D)** right CC mammograms. On the current exam, the oval mass (*arrow*) at the 7 o'clock position is similar in size, but there has been a subtle change in the shape of the mass: the current mass appears more lobulated than the previous one.

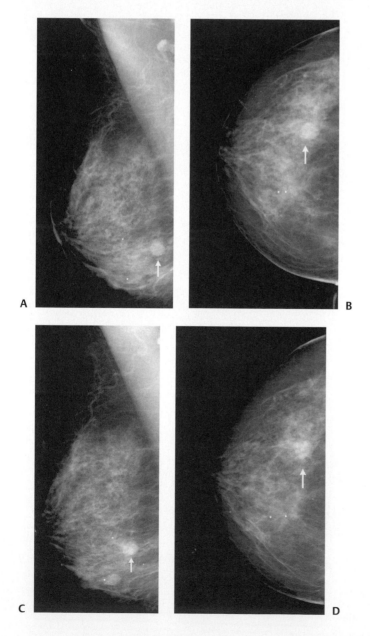

A   B

C   D

Ultrasonography

Figure 6–18 (E) Right breast sonogram and **(F)** right color Doppler sonogram performed 2 years prior to the current exam. This sonogram was performed for a new oval mass at the 7 o'clock position. The mammographic mass corresponded to a solid hypoechoic mildly lobulated mass. This mass exhibited increased color flow Doppler **(D)**. **(G)** Right breast sonogram. This ultrasound was performed following the mammograms in **(C)** and **(D)**. At the 7 o'clock position, there is still a solid hypoechoic mass. Sonographically, this mass is similar in size to the previous exam, but it has changed in appearance. The margins are irregular in shape.

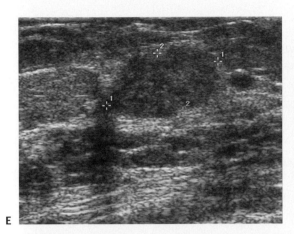

E

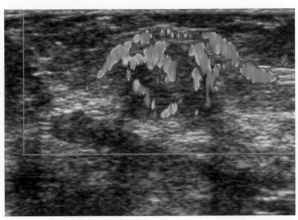

F

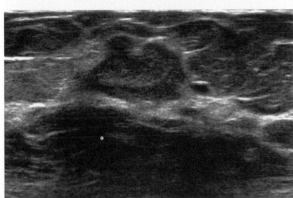

G

Management   BI-RADS category 4, suspicious. Biopsy should be considered.

Pathologic Diagnosis

Malignant

Intracystic papillary carcinoma

Pearls and Pitfalls

- Solid masses that have well-defined borders and oval or gently lobulated shapes should be assessed as category 3, probably benign, with recommended short-term follow-up. Generally, these lesions should be closely followed for 2 years before sending the patient back to the screening pool.

■ Case 6–19

Characteristics of Masses   Irregular masses

Clinical History   A 48-year-old woman presents with a left breast lump.

Physical Examination   Left breast: Palpable lump at the 10 o'clock position near the areola.

Radiologic Findings

Mammography

Figure 6–19 Mediolateral oblique (MLO) and craniocaudal (CC) views. **(A)** Left MLO and **(B)** left CC mammograms. There is an irregular mass (*arrows*) in the upper inner quadrant.

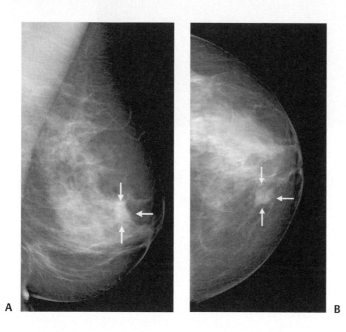

A   B

Ultrasonography

Figure 6–19 (C) Left breast sonogram. The palpable mammographic mass corresponds to a hypoechoic mass with ill-defined, irregular lobulated margins.

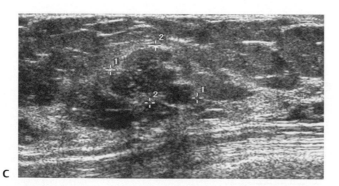

C

Management   BI-RADS category 4, suspicious. Biopsy should be considered.

Pathologic Diagnosis

Benign

Fibroadenoma

Pearls and Pitfalls

- Because fibroadenomas are so common, they frequently present mammographically as an irregular mass. Sonography generally does not reduce the suspiciousness of these lesions, and they should be biopsied.

■ Case 6–20

Characteristics of Masses   Irregular masses

Clinical History   A 51-year-old woman presents for screening.

Physical Examination   Normal exam

Radiologic Findings

Mammography

Figure 6–20 Mediolateral (ML) views. **(A)** Right ML mammogram. **(B)** Right spot magnification ML mammogram. In the upper outer quadrant, there is an irregular mass (*arrows*).

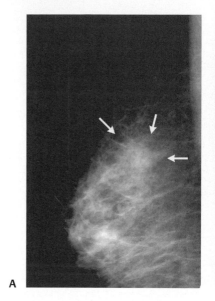
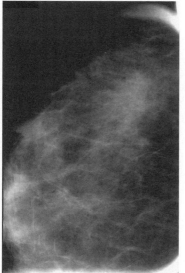
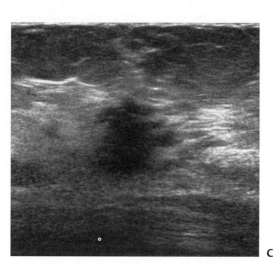

Figure 6–20 (C) Right breast sonogram. In the upper outer quadrant, the mammographic mass corresponds to a solid irregular hypoechoic mass.

Ultrasonography

Management   BI-RADS category 4, suspicious. Biopsy should be considered.

Pathologic Diagnosis

Malignant

Ductal carcinoma in situ (DCIS)

Pearls and Pitfalls

- In ~10% of cases, DCIS presents as a mammographic soft tissue mass without calcifications. In this circumstance, the mammographic and sonographic findings are similar to the invasive malignancies.

■ Case 6–21

Characteristics of Masses   Irregular masses

Clinical History   A 61-year-old woman presents with a left palpable mass.

Physical Examination   Right breast: Normal exam. Left breast: Lump at the 10 o'clock position.

Radiologic Findings

Mammography

Figure 6–21 Mediolateral oblique (MLO) and craniocaudal (CC) views. **(A)** Left MLO spot compression. **(B)** Left CC spot compression (10 o'clock mass). **(C)** Left CC spot compression (12 o'clock mass). There are two irregular spiculated masses at 10 and 12 o'clock.

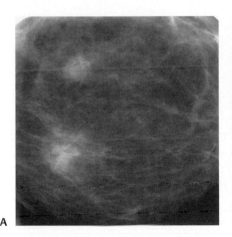
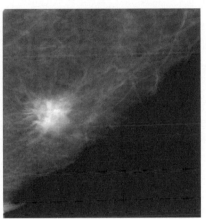
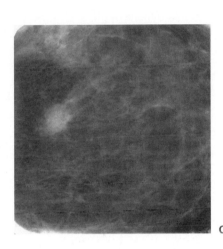

A   B   C

Ultrasonography

Figure 6–21 **(D)** Left breast sonogram (10 o'clock) and **(E)** left breast sonogram (12 o'clock). The spiculated mammographic masses correspond to two irregular hypoechoic solid masses. The 10 o'clock mass is the palpable one.

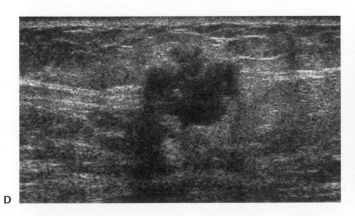
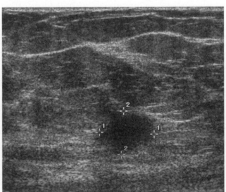

D   E

Management BI-RADS category 5, highly suggestive of malignancy

Pathologic Diagnosis

Malignant

Infiltrating ductal carcinoma

Comments on Histology Both masses are infiltrating ductal carcinoma.

Pearls and Pitfalls

- The mammographic appearances of the masses are highly suspicious for malignancy (category 5). The sonogram is performed to localize for biopsy; this exam is not necessary for assessment.

■ Case 6–22

Characteristics of Masses   Irregular masses

Clinical History   A 65-year-old woman notes a left breast lump.

Physical Examination   Left breast: Lump at the 2 o'clock position.

Radiologic Findings

Mammography

Figure 6–22 Mediolateral oblique (MLO) and craniocaudal (CC) views. **(A)** Left MLO, **(B)** left CC, **(C)** left MLO spot compression, and **(D)** left CC spot compression mammograms. In the upper outer breast, there is an irregular mass.

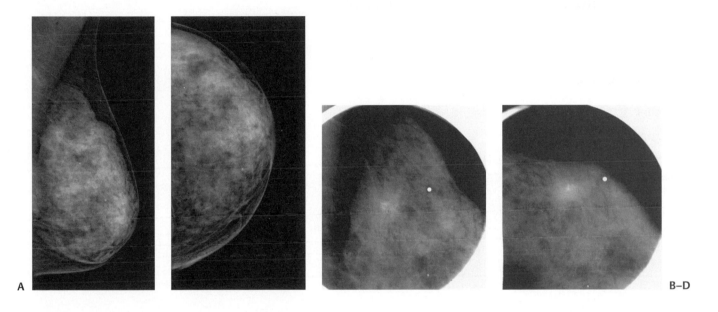

Ultrasonography

Figure 6–22 (E) Left breast sonogram. The palpable mammographic mass corresponds to an irregular hypoechoic solid mass.

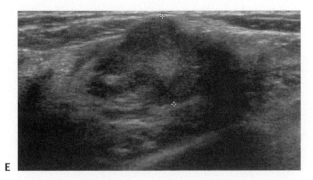

Magnetic Resonance Imaging

Figure 6–22 (F) Bilateral breast MRI (subtraction series: 2 minutes after injection of contrast). There is a solitary enhancing mass in the upper outer quadrant. No other masses or adenopathy is identified.

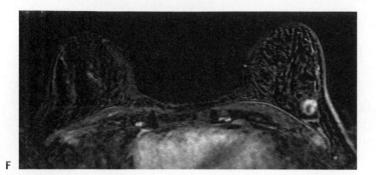

F

Management   BI-RADS category 4, suspicious. Biopsy should be considered.

Pathologic Diagnosis

Malignant

Infiltrating ductal carcinoma

Pearls and Pitfalls

- This exam demonstrates the utility of digital mammography in women with dense breasts. Multiple studies have shown that when patients receive both digital and screen-film mammograms, mammographers judge that the patients' breasts are less dense with digital mammography than with screen-film mammography.

■ Case 6–23

Characteristics of Masses　Irregular masses

Clinical History　A 73-year-old woman presents for screening.

Physical Examination　Normal exam

Radiologic Findings

Mammography

Figure 6–23 Mediolateral oblique (MLO) and craniocaudal (CC) views. (**A**) Left MLO, (**B**) left CC, and (**C**) left CC spot magnification mammograms. In the upper inner quadrant, there is a small mass (*arrow*). On spot magnification, the mass has microlobulated margins.

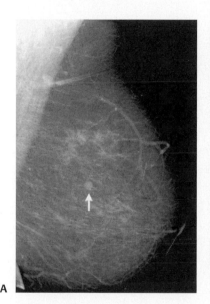
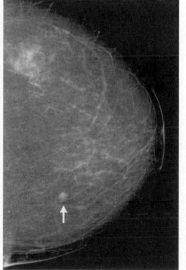
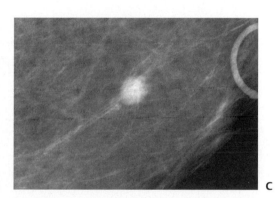

A　　　　　　　　　　B　　　　　　　　　　C

Ultrasonography

Figure 6–23 (**D**) Left breast sonogram. At the 10 o'clock position, the mammographic mass corresponds to an irregular hypoechoic solid mass with a thick echogenic halo.

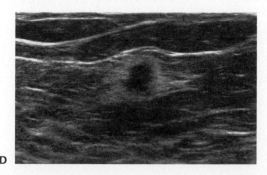

D

Management   BI-RADS category 5, highly suggestive of malignancy

Pathologic Diagnosis

Malignant

Infiltrating ductal carcinoma

Pearls and Pitfalls

- This case demonstrates that small masses benefit from digital mammographic spot magnification imaging. The magnification technique reveals the irregular microlobulated margins of the mass.

■ Case 6–24

Characteristics of Masses   Irregular masses

Clinical History   A 52-year-old woman presents with a left breast lump.

Physical Examination   Left breast: Large mass involving most of the upper outer quadrant.

Radiologic Findings

Mammography

Figure 6–24 Mediolateral oblique (MLO) and craniocaudal (CC) views. **(A)** Left MLO, **(B)** left CC, **(C)** left MLO spot compression, and **(D)** left CC spot compression mammograms. In the upper outer quadrant, there is an irregular mass. Adjacent to this dominant mass is a smaller oval circumscribed mass that is suspicious for an abnormal intramammary node. Axillary adenopathy is also present.

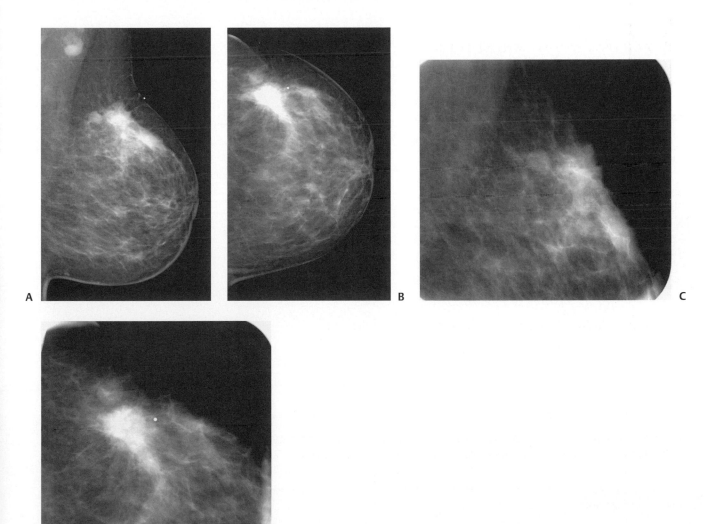

Ultrasonography

Figure 6–24 (E) Left breast sonogram. The palpable mammographic mass corresponds to a large hypoechoic irregular mass. Adjacent to this mass is a smaller oval mass consistent with a small lymph node.

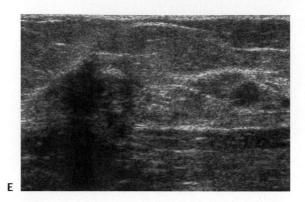

E

Magnetic Resonance Imaging

Figure 6–24 (F) Bilateral breast MRI (subtraction series: 2 minutes after injection of contrast). There is a large enhancing irregular mass associated with enhancing axillary adenopathy.

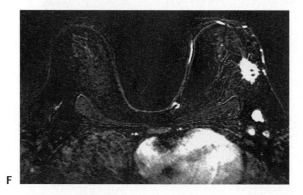

F

Management   BI-RADS category 5, highly suggestive of malignancy

Pathologic Diagnosis

Malignant

Infiltrating ductal carcinoma

Comments on Histology   Left mastectomy: Three of 14 nodes exhibited metastatic disease. One intramammary node was positive for metastatic disease.

Pearls and Pitfalls

- Axillary nodal involvement with breast cancer is an important prognostic factor in survival. Survival rates decrease with an increasing number of positive nodes. For example, patients with tumors smaller than 2 cm have 5-year survival rates of 96.3% with negative nodes, 87.4% with one to three positive nodes, and 66% with four or more positive nodes.

■ Case 6–25

Characteristics of Masses   Irregular masses

Clinical History   A 66-year-old woman presents for screening. She originally received a screen-film exam because her breasts were too large for the digital plates. An ill-defined left breast mass was identified at the 9 o'clock position. Left breast sonography demonstrated a highly suspicious mass (category 5). However, this sonographic mass could not be localized when she returned for biopsy. The patient's mass was then biopsied using the stereotaxic technique.

Physical Examination   Normal exam

Radiologic Findings

Mammography

Figure 6–25 Mediolateral oblique (MLO) and craniocaudal (CC) views. **(A)** Left MLO and **(B)** left CC mammograms. These digital images are performed to localize the irregular mass (*square*) at the 9 o'clock position prior to stereotaxic biopsy. **(C)** Left CC needle localization mammogram. The biopsied malignant mass now has a clip from the prior biopsy.

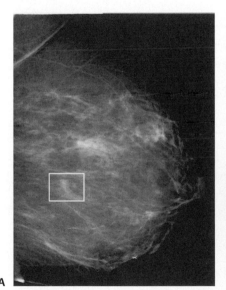
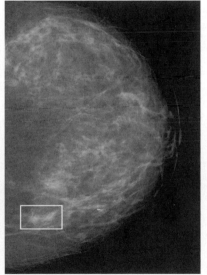
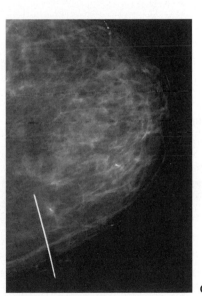

A

B

C

Ultrasonography

Figure 6–25 (D) Left breast sonogram. At the 9 o'clock position, there is an irregular hypoechoic mass with a thick echogenic halo. The small size of the mass (8 mm), the long distance from the nipple (10 cm), and the large breast size contributed to the failure to identify this mass when the patient returned for biopsy.

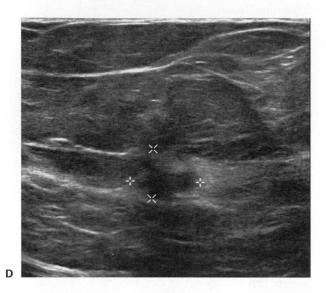

D

Management   BI-RADS category 4, suspicious. Biopsy should be considered.

Pathologic Diagnosis

Malignant

Infiltrating ductal carcinoma

Pearls and Pitfalls

- This case illustrates that even if the patient's breasts are too large for the screening compression plates, digital mammography is an ideal technology for interventional applications. When performing interventional procedures, only a small area of the breast is needed for imaging. When placing the needle for biopsy, the digital localization images can be viewed quickly, unlike film, which must be processed.

■ Case 6–26

Characteristics of Masses   Circumscribed masses

Clinical History   A 76-year-old woman is found to have a new right mammographic mass.

Physical Examination   Normal exam

Radiologic Findings

Mammography

Figure 6–26 Mediolateral oblique (MLO) and craniocaudal (CC) views. **(A)** Right MLO spot compression and **(B)** right CC spot compression mammograms. There is a well-circumscribed lobulated mass in the inner, inferior breast.

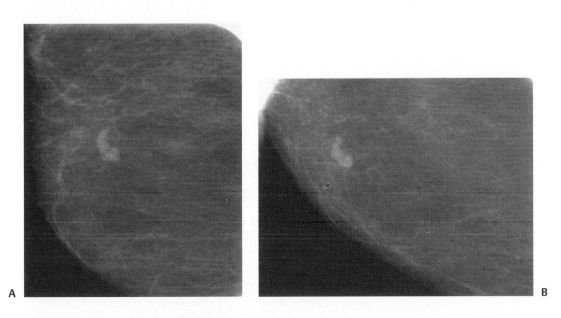

A   B

Ultrasonography

Figure 6–26 (C) Right breast sonogram. The mammographic mass corresponds to a lobulated mass with mildly angulated margins.

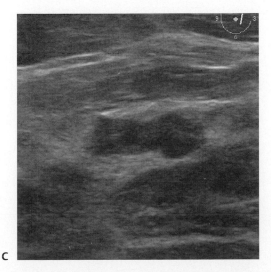

C

Management   BI-RADS category 4, suspicious. Biopsy should be considered.

Pathologic Diagnosis

Malignant

Invasive papillary carcinoma

Pearls and Pitfalls

- Invasive papillary carcinoma comprises only ~2% of all invasive cancers.

■ Case 6–27

Characteristics of Masses   Irregular masses

Clinical History   A 46-year-old woman presents to the emergency room with chest pain. Computed tomography, chest: Left breast mass and T5 vertebral body metastasis.

Physical Examination   Left breast: There is a palpable lump at the 9 o'clock position. The skin of the medial breast is warm, slightly red, and thickened, characteristic of peau d'orange. The nipple is inverted.

Radiologic Findings

Mammography

Figure 6–27 Mediolateral oblique (MLO) and craniocaudal (CC) views. **(A)** Left MLO and **(B)** left CC mammograms. At the 9 o'clock position, there is an irregular mass associated with skin thickening and nipple inversion.

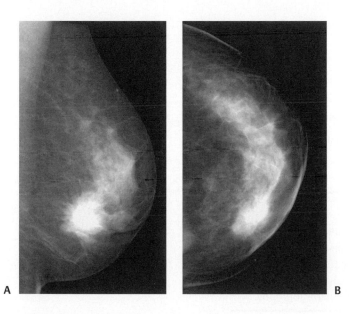

A   B

Ultrasonography

Figure 6–27 **(C)** Left radial and **(D)** left antiradial breast sonograms. At the 9 o'clock position, the mammographically palpable mass corresponds to an irregular mass of heterogeneous echogenicity. The mass extends to the nipple (N). Skin thickening (S) is also evident adjacent to the mass.

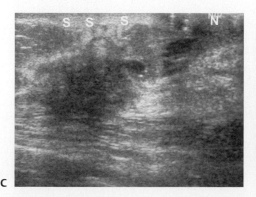

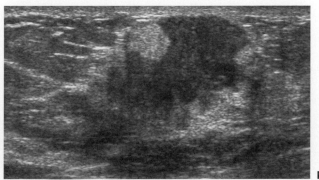

C   D

Magnetic Resonance Imaging

Figure 6–27 (E) Bilateral breast MRI (subtraction image: 2 minutes after contrast injection). There is rapid malignant enhancement of the 9 o'clock left breast mass as well as the adjacent skin. **(F)** Bilateral breast MRI (subtraction image: 2 minutes after contrast injection). In the same study as **E,** abnormal axillary lymphadenopathy is identified (*arrow*).

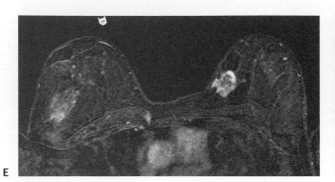
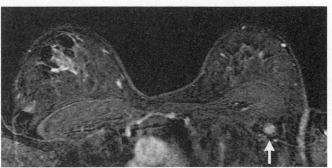

E   F

Management   BI-RADS category 5, highly suggestive of malignancy

Pathologic Diagnosis

Malignant

Inflammatory carcinoma

Comments on Histology   Histology of the primary malignancy in this case is infiltrating ductal carcinoma.

Pearls and Pitfalls

- Mammographic findings of inflammatory breast cancer include skin thickening (>90%), increased breast density (<90%), trabecular thickening (85%), and nipple inversion (~50%). Digital mammography has the potential to improve the display of inflammatory cancer because manipulation of the display allows for better visualization of the nipple and skin compared with screen-film mammography.

■ Case 6–28

Characteristics of Masses   Irregular masses

History   A 37-year-old woman presents initially having noticed left breast skin changes 1 year ago. Since that time her skin thickening has worsened.

Physical Examination   Left breast: Diffuse skin thickening, warmth, and redness (peau d'orange). No palpable mass.

Radiologic Findings

Mammography

Figure 6–28 Mediolateral oblique (MLO) and craniocaudal (CC) views. **(A)** Left MLO, **(B)** left CC, **(C)** and left CC magnification mammograms. There is diffuse increased density with skin thickening. At the 6 o'clock position, there is an irregular mass with coarse heterogeneous calcifications distributed in a linear branching pattern. There is a second ill-defined, irregular mass in the upper outer quadrant.

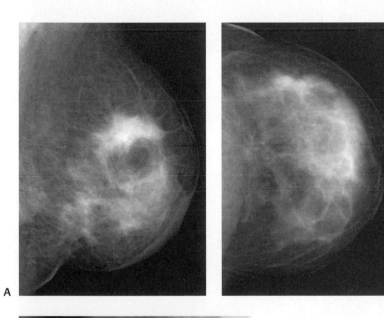

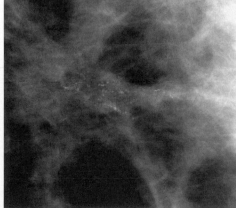

Ultrasonography

Figure 6–28 (D) Left breast sonogram at 6 o'clock. There is an irregular hypoechoic solid mass that corresponds to the mammographic mass with calcifications. **(E)** Left breast sonogram at 2 o'clock. There is an irregular hypoechoic mass that corresponds to the mammographic mass in the upper outer quadrant. This mass is extending through Cooper's ligament (*arrows*) to the skin, which is diffusely thickened.

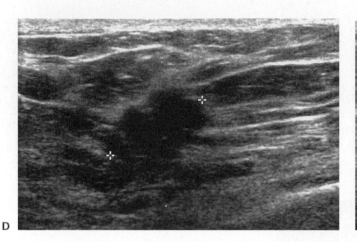

D

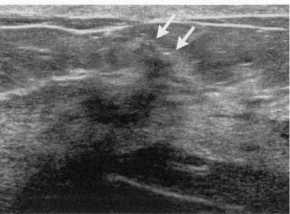

E

Magnetic Resonance Imaging

Figure 6–28 (F) Bilateral breast MRI (subtraction image: 2 minutes after contrast injection). This image demonstrates the rapid abnormal contrast enhancement associated with the 2 o'clock mass. There is also diffuse skin thickening. Besides the two malignant masses, this MRI exam identifies axillary adenopathy (at a different transverse level), later confirmed to represent metastatic disease.

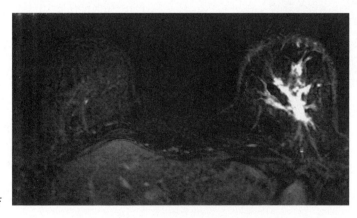

F

Management   BI-RADS category 5, highly suggestive of malignancy

Pathologic Diagnosis

Malignant

Inflammatory carcinoma

Comments on Histology   The histology of the 6 o'clock mass is infiltrating ductal carcinoma. The histology of the 2 o'clock mass is infiltrating lobular carcinoma.

Pearls and Pitfalls

- Inflammatory breast cancer represents between 1 and 2% of all breast cancers. About one third of patients may present without a mass. In these cases, the main differential diagnosis is mastitis. Therefore, careful mammographic evaluation for masses or suspicious calcifications is important for women with prolonged evidence of inflammatory breast symptoms.

7 Digital Mammographic Technique for Mammographic Asymmetries

There are relatively limited data concerning the appearance of asymmetries on digital compared with screen-film mammography. The studies examining patients with both techniques have shown no significant difference in the identification of malignant asymmetries.[1,2] The most common reason for discrepancies for all malignant assessments included fortuitous positioning and differences in diagnostic opinions.[1] Because asymmetries tend to be more subtle than masses or calcifications, patient positioning may affect visualization of asymmetries more than these other lesions. However, neither positioning nor diagnostic opinion differentiates digital from screen-film technique.

▪ General Evaluation of Mammographic Asymmetries

Asymmetries differ from masses in that they do not appear to have a three-dimensional volume. They lack convex borders, usually contain interspersed fat, and do not have a consistent shape in orthogonal planes.[3] Asymmetries appear to represent a relative increase in the volume of fibroglandular tissue of the affected area compared with the contralateral region.[4] Commonly, they are visible only on one screening view. There are two types of asymmetries: global and focal. Global asymmetries involve at least one quarter of a breast and are not palpable. About 3% of women have asymmetrical fibroglandular composition with symmetric breast volume.[5] If global asymmetry represents asymmetry of normal fibroglandular tissue, then the tissue should have the same characteristics as normal fibroglandular tissue. The tissue lacks a specific shape. The area consists of curvilinear lines with interspersed fat. There are no convex borders or margins.

Although some patients have asymmetric fibroglandular composition on their baseline exams, other patients develop global asymmetries with increasing age. Overall, fibroglandular composition commonly decreases with age and is associated with reduction in endogenous estrogen. This normal reduction in fibroglandular composition may result in either global or focal asymmetries.

Besides physiologic causes for global asymmetry, medications may affect breast composition and produce global asymmetries. For example, hormone replacement therapy promotes estrogen effect on the breast and may increase fibroglandular composition.[6,7]

If the global asymmetry involves skin thickening, then one should consider etiologies such as axillary lymphatic obstruction, lymphatic spread of breast cancer, inflammation, postradiation effect, and systemic fluid overload.[8] Axillary lymphatic obstruction results from surgical removal of axillary lymph nodes or is produced by malignancies such as metastatic axillary breast cancer and hematologic malignancies that block lymphatic drainage. Breast cancer sometimes metastasizes via lymphatic spread to the contralateral breast and produces lymphatic obstruction and lymphedema. Besides lymphatic obstruction, skin thickening may be caused by excess fluid or edema. Abscess with associated inflammation will produce skin thickening. Because abscesses are commonly subareolar, the skin thickening and increased density are primarily around the areola and decrease toward the axilla. Finally, systemic fluid overload from etiologies such as congestive heart failure and renal failure may produce skin thickening.

Because factors outside the breast commonly produce global asymmetries, the work-up of global asymmetries should include a good patient history that covers any personal history of breast cancer. Because of hormone therapy's influence on the breast, this information should be included on the clinical questionnaire administered to patients prior to mammographic examination. If the patient is symptomatic, then the patient's symptoms should be recorded. If skin thickening is present, then the patient should be questioned about personal history of malignancy, infection, and illnesses producing systemic fluid overload. If the patient is new to the mammographic facility, she should be questioned about availability of previous examinations, as comparison with earlier mammographic examinations are particularly useful to assess stability of asymmetry. If the global asymmetry is new, and the asymmetry cannot be identified as normal fibroglandular tissue or ascribed to a known etiology, then this asymmetry should be evaluated using the same methods as a focal asymmetry.

Focal asymmetries are smaller than global asymmetries. With high-contrast digital postprocessing, focal asymmetries are frequently visible. Comparison with previous examinations is important to determine if the asymmetry is a developing density. Because asymmetries are difficult to differentiate from surrounding fibroglandular tissue in more than one view, malignancies that appear in this manner tend to be the most difficult ones to detect. Like global asymmetry, the focal asymmetry is evaluated to determine if it is normal asymmetric fibroglandular tissue or a mass. Besides lacking defined shape, margins, and conspicuity, normal fibroglandular tissue consists of curvilinear lines interspersed with tiny islands of fat that are directed to the nipple. If the asymmetry is on the periphery, the edges of the asymmetry gradually fade in a feathery pattern into the surrounding fat. One should evaluate the asymmetry for associated factors that strongly suggest the presence of a mass such as architectural distortion, calcifications, or associated palpable lump.

If a focal asymmetry is suspicious, the lesion should be characterized and localized. Spot compression mammography applied on a focal asymmetry can confirm the presence of a mass by clarifying the shape, margins, and position of the abnormality.[9,10] However, spot compression has several weaknesses, including poor characterization of subtle masses and poor localization of masses visible only in one view. Furthermore, spot compression requires a technologist with skilled mammographic technique.

Masses that initially appear as focal asymmetries tend to be subtle. This subtle appearance may be due to small size, obscuration of the mass by dense surrounding fibroglandular tissue, or increased compressibility. If the asymmetry represents a small mass surrounded by fibroglandular tissue, compression of the mass may not separate it from the surrounding density. If the asymmetry is compressible, as with some lobular carcinomas, then the lesion may not be visible with spot compression views because it will be "pressed out."

Besides inadequately characterizing subtle masses, spot compression views may not effectively localize focal asymmetries visible in only one screening view. In these cases, multiple spot compression views may need to be performed to identify the lesion. Many times, even after multiple attempts, the asymmetry is not clearly identified on an orthogonal view.

The final disadvantage of spot compression views is that this technique is operator dependent. Although digital mammography allows for more flexibility in imaging parameters, for subtle lesions, the mammography technologist should place the mass in the middle of the spot compression field for optimal visualization. This placement may not be difficult when the asymmetry is easily visible. However, if the asymmetry is subtle or visible in only one view, then placement of a poorly visible asymmetry is difficult.

Other techniques used to evaluate focal asymmetries are alternative localizing views (90 degrees, either mediolateral [ML] or lateromedial [LM] and exaggerated craniocaudal [XCCL] views), rolled craniocaudal (CC) views, and shallow mediolateral oblique (MLO) views. If the location of the focal asymmetry is clear, then the ML or LM and XCCL views are useful to further localize the asymmetry for future sonographic evaluation or biopsy.

If the location of the focal asymmetry is not clear, then either the rolled CC or shallow MLO views can be used to localize the lesion. With the rolled CC technique (**Fig. 7–1**), the breast is placed in the CC position on the mammographic unit. Prior to compressing the breast, the top of the breast is rolled medially (so that the bottom of the breast is rolled laterally). The breast is then compressed in this "rolled" position. If the lesion is in the superior half of the breast, it will move medially. If the lesion is in the inferior half of the breast, it will move laterally. After the image has been taken, the breast is then uncompressed and brought back to the neutral position. The breast is then rolled in the opposite position—the superior breast rolls laterally, and the inferior breast rolls medially. Lesions in the superior breast will then move laterally, and those in the inferior breast will move medially. Images must be labeled so that the direction the breast was rolled is recorded (**Fig. 7–1**).[5,11]

The localization method preferred by the author is the shallow oblique technique (**Fig. 7–2**). This technique is particularly useful when the asymmetry is identified in only one view, and there is concern that it is a subtle mass. In this technique, the first step is to determine the screening view in which the asymmetry is best identified. Next, MLO images are done at 10 and 20 degrees from the original view. The angles chosen for the oblique views are designed to (1) be slightly different from the original view and (2) provide smaller incremental steps closer to the other screening view. For example, if the lesion is best identified in the CC (0-degree) view, then MLO views are done at 10 and 20 degrees. If the lesion is best identified on the 60-degree MLO view, then MLO views are done at 50 and 40 degrees. The four images—original MLO, two shallow MLOs, and original CC—are aligned in a row, with the nipples at the same horizontal level. The asymmetry is then identified in each view. Referring to the latter example when the asymmetry is visible only on the 60-degree MLO view, the three MLO views (60-, 50-, 40-degrees) are close to each other in position; there is only a slight shift in the overall parenchymal pattern with each view. Generally, the asymmetry can be identified in these three MLO views. Once the asymmetry has been identified in the three MLO views, the position of the asymmetry can be extrapolated in the fourth view (**Table 7–1**).[11,12] This table summarizes the method to localize asymmetries which are initially only visible in one view. As an example, reviewing the top line: if the asymmetry is only visible on the lateral aspect of the CC view and appears to stay above the nipple on two successive oblique views, then the lesion will be in the upper breast on the MLO view or in the upper outer qudrant. In order to best apply this method, one should also observe changes in the surrounding parenchymal position compared to the lesion. Although this method works in most cases, in cases in which there is a large change in relative lesion position with each shallow oblique, the final lesion position may be on the opposite side of the nipple from the expected position. However, these exceptions can be identified if the observer notices the change in the relative position of the lesion compared to the surrounding fibroglandular parenchymal pattern. Using this system for localizing asymmetries, the radiologist would use the guidelines outlined in **Table 7–2** to determine the Breast Imaging Reporting and Data System (BI-RADS) category.

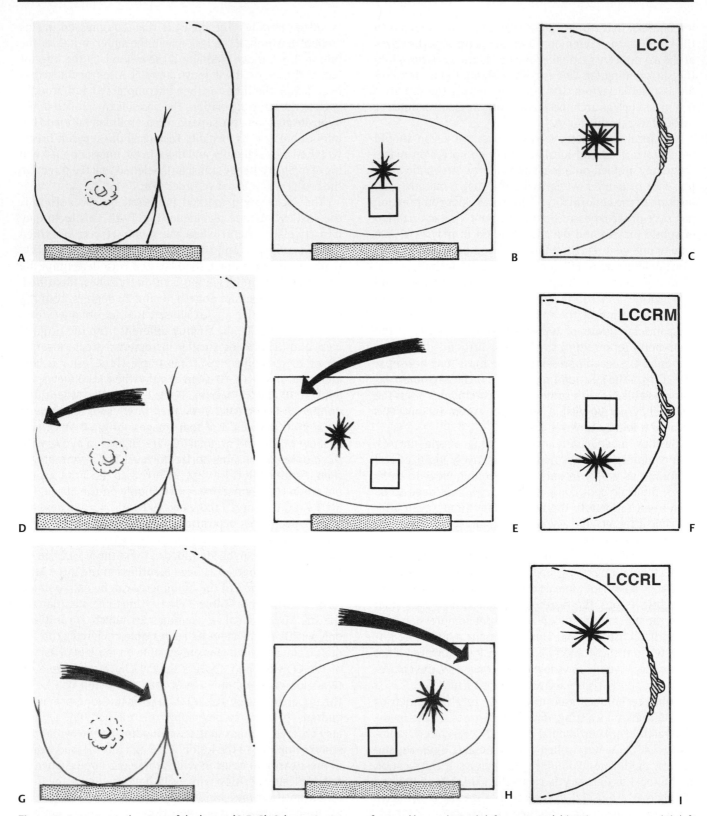

Figure 7–1 Anatomic drawings of the breast **(A,D,G)**. Schematic pictures of coronal breast **(B,E,H)**, left craniocaudal (LCC) mammogram **(C)**, left craniocaudal rolled medial (LCCRM) mammogram **(F)**, left craniocaudal rolled lateral (LCCRL) mammogram **(I)**.

    (A–C) Neutral position. In the neutral position, the spiculated mass and the square asymmetry are overlapping in the LCC view. **(D–F)** Rolled medial CC. When the breast is rolled medially, the anterior spiculated mass moves medially, and the posterior square asymmetry moves laterally. Therefore, in the LCCRM view, the spiculated mass is medial to the square asymmetry. **(G–I)** Rolled lateral CC. When the breast is rolled laterally, the anterior spiculated mass moves laterally and the posterior square asymmetry moves medially. As a result, the spiculated mass is lateral to the square asymmetry in the LCCRL.

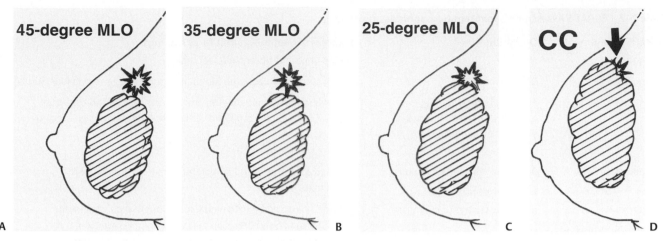

Figure 7–2 Shallow oblique views for localization. The lesion initially is identified only on the mediolateral oblique (MLO) view superior to the nipple. **(A)** The screening MLO is performed at 45 degrees. Therefore, the **(B)** 35- and **(C)** 25-degree MLO views are performed first, then placed between the original 45-degree MLO and the **(D)** craniocaudal (CC) view. The lesion in the oblique views appears to remain above the nipple. Therefore, in the CC view **(D)**, the lesion is in the upper outer quadrant. In retrospect, the spiculated mass (*arrow*) is identified partially obscured by adjacent fibroglandular tissue.

The advantage of the shallow MLO views is that they are operator independent, requiring only a mammography technologist to perform them. For lesions that are compressible, the use of a wider field of view compression device is less likely to overcompress a mass. This method localizes an asymmetry for sonographic examination of the lesion or for biopsy of the abnormality. The major disadvantage of this technique depends on the flexibility of the digital workstation to place the images adjacent to each other.

The assessment of asymmetries is one of the greatest challenges of mammography. With the increasing application of sonography and magnetic resonance and the increasing fear of medicolegal repercussions, breast imagers have become more aware of the presence of mammographically subtle or occult breast neoplasms.[13–15] Many of these neoplasms appear mammographically as asymmetries. This awareness has resulted in more aggressive work-up of asymmetries. However, the drive to identify these subtle cancers is balanced by the necessity to limit the harm caused by the number of false-positive mammographic assessments.[16] In logically approaching the work-up of asymmetries, one should have an objective method (**Table 7–2**).

The author has found the following approach useful in guiding the work-up and assessment of asymmetries. When identifying an asymmetry, first decide if the asymmetry represents the same volume of density or an increase

Table 7–1 Method to Determine Location with Shallow Oblique Views

Screening View Lesion Visible	Position of Lesion in Screening View	Location of Lesion in Shallow Obliques	Lesion Location/Quadrant
CC	Lateral breast	Stays above nipple	Upper outer quadrant
CC	Lateral breast	Moves below nipple	Lower outer quadrant
CC	Medial breast	Moves above nipple	Upper medial quadrant
CC	Medial breast	Stays below nipple	Lower medial quadrant
MLO	Superior breast	Stays above nipple	Upper outer quadrant
MLO	Superior breast	Moves below nipple	Upper medial quadrant
MLO	Inferior breast	Moves above nipple	Lower outer quadrant
MLO	Inferior breast	Stays below nipple	Lower medial quadrant

Table 7–1 This table summarizes the method to localize asymmetries which are initially only visible in one view. As an example, reviewing the top line: if the asymmetry is only visible on the lateral aspect of the CC view and appears to stay above the nipple on 2 successive oblique views, then the lesion will be in the upper breast on the MLO view or in upper outer quadrant. In order to best apply this method, one should also observe changes in the surrounding parenchymal position compared to the lesion. Although this method works in most cases, in cases where there is a large change in relative lesion position with each shallow oblique, the final lesion position may be on the opposite side of the nipple from the expected position. However, these exceptions can be identified if the observer notices the change in the relative position of the lesion compared to the surrounding fibroglandular parenchymal pattern. *CC*, craniocaudal; MLO, mediolateral oblique.

Table 7–2   BI-RADS Assessments for Mammographic Asymmetries

BI-RADS Assessment	Definition	Examples of Mammographic Mass Findings
Category 1	Negative	Overlap of normal fibroglandular tissue
Category 2	Benign finding	Normal fibroglandular tissue (no change in volume since previous exams)
Category 3	Probably benign finding; initial short-term interval follow-up suggested	Normal fibroglandular tissue (no previous exam or possible relative increase in volume compared with contralateral side since previous exams) Negative sonogram
Category 4	Suspicious abnormality; biopsy should be considered	Developing density; irregular mammographic or sonographic solid mass
Category 5	Highly suspicious of malignancy	Asymmetry associated with highly suspicious malignant findings (architectural distortion, skin thickening, nipple inversion, trabecular thickening, skin retraction, or malignant microcalcifications)

BI-RADS, Breast Imaging Reporting and Data System.

in the volume of density compared with the previous exam or, if no previous exam is available, the contralateral side. Second, using spot compression, rolled views, or shallow obliques, localize and characterize the asymmetry. These techniques should provide sufficient information about the internal structure, shape, and location of the asymmetry. Third, determine if there is any sign of a mass: any faint irregular margins, architectural distortion, or microcalcifications. The mass may be subtle, so if the asymmetry persists in only one of the additional views, a mass should be suspected. When evaluating an asymmetry, it is important to aggressively evaluate previous exams, as increasing density (i.e., developing density) over time is an indication that the finding should be worked up. If the asymmetry appears to represent normal fibroglandular tissue, then it is assessed as category 1, negative or BI-RADS category 2, benign finding. The author reserves these categories for patients in which the asymmetry represents normal fibroglandular tissue that has not changed in volume compared with previous exams. The most common reasons for these asymmetries are differences in compression, patient position, and imaging parameters.

The author has a separate group of asymmetries that are assessed as BI-RADS category 3, probably benign. These asymmetries also appear to be normal fibroglandular tissue; however, unlike the BI-RADS category 2 group, category 3 may represent an increase in the relative volume of fibroglandular tissue and, therefore, may correspond to neodensities or developing densities. Common reasons for this situation are when the patient has no previous comparison exams (e.g., the asymmetry is on a baseline exam) and when the asymmetry appears to be due to a normal explainable cause, such as asymmetric involution of fibroglandular tissue with age. With this group, the author always sonographically examines the area of the

asymmetry to eliminate any subtle neoplasm. If the sonogram is negative, then the patient is assessed as BI-RADS category 3, probably benign finding, with an initial short-interval follow-up suggested. In this case, the author recommends a 6-month follow-up unilateral mammogram. If that mammogram is stable, then the patient has bilateral mammograms 6 months and 1 year later.

The reason for separating this group of asymmetries for short-term follow-up is that, within this group, increasing volume of normal fibroglandular tissue is commonly difficult to separate from the potentially malignant developing densities. Retrospectively, this is one of the most common perceptual errors in assessing asymmetries. Rosen et al note that 10 of 12 (83%) asymmetries missed in their series were actually developing densities.[17] They and other researchers suggest that sonography is useful but have not delineated specific guidelines concerning sonographic applications to mammographic asymmetries.[17,18] The author concurs that sonography is extremely useful in guiding assessment of these difficult lesions, but one major problem in applying sonography is that asymmetries are often difficult to localize mammographically. If the imager is unsure of the location of the asymmetry, sonography has limited benefit. Therefore, prior to proceeding to sonography, a complete mammographic work-up, including localization of the asymmetry, is crucial.

Finally, if the diagnostic mammographic or sonographic imaging demonstrates evidence that the asymmetry is a developing density or suspicious mass, the asymmetry is assessed as BI-RADS category 4, suspicious. Sonography may be used for biopsy guidance. Asymmetries that are associated with obvious signs of malignancy (e.g., skin thickening, nipple inversion, malignant calcifications, and architectural distortion) are assessed as category 5, highly suggestive of malignancy.

References

1. Lewin JM, D'Orsi CJ, Hendrick RE. Clinical comparison of full-field digital mammography and screen-film mammography for detection of breast cancer. Am J Roentgenol 2002;179:671–677
2. Venta LA, Hendrick RE, Adler YT. Rates and causes of disagreement in interpretation of full-field digital mammography and film-screen mammography in a diagnostic setting. Am J Roentgenol 2001;176:1241–1248
3. Sickles EA. Breast masses: mammographic evaluation. Radiology 1989;173:297–303
4. Fu KL, Fu YS, Bassett LW, Cardall SY, Lopez JK. Invasive malignancies. In: Bassett LW, Jackson VP, Fu KL, Fu YS, eds. Diagnosis of Diseases of the Breast. Philadelphia: Elsevier Saunders; 2005: 438–517
5. Ikeda DM. Mammogram interpretation. In: Breast Imaging: The Requisites. Philadelphia: Elsevier Mosby; 2004:24–59
6. Cyrlak D, Wong CH. Mammographic changes in postmenopausal women undergoing hormonal replacement therapy. Am J Roentgenol 1993;161:1177–1183
7. Laya MB, Gallagher JC, Schreiman JS, Larson EB, Watson P, Weinstein L. Effect of postmenopausal hormonal replacement therapy on mammographic density and parenchymal pattern. Radiology 1995;196:433–437
8. Tabar L, Dean PB. Thickened skin syndrome of the breast. In: Tabar L, Dean PB, eds. Teaching Atlas of Mammography. New York: Thieme Medical Publishers; 2001:239–247
9. Tabar L, Dean PB, Tot T. Mammographic-histologic correlation of tumor masses, asymmetric densities and architectural distortion. In: Feig SA, ed. Breast Imaging. Oak Brook, IL: RSNA; 2005:9–29
10. Berkowitz JE, Gatewood OMB, Gayler BW. Equivocal mammographic findings: evaluation with spot compression. Radiology 1989;171:369–371
11. Sickles EA. Practical solutions to common mammographic problems: tailoring the examination. Am J Roentgenol 1988;151:31–39
12. Pearson KL, Sickles EA, Frankel SD, Leung JW. Efficacy of step-oblique mammography for confirmation and localization of densities seen on only one standard mammographic view. Am J Roentgenol 2000;174:745–752
13. Ikeda DM, Andersson I, Wattsgard C, Janzon L, Linell F. Interval carcinomas in the Malmö mammographic screening trial: radiographic appearance and prognostic considerations. Am J Roentgenol 1992;159:287–294
14. Harvey JA, Fajardo LL, Innis CA. Previous mammograms in patients with impalpable breast carcinoma: retrospective vs. blinded interpretation. AJR Am J Roentgenol 1993;161:1167–1172
15. Ikeda DM, Birdwell RL, O'Shaughnessy KF, Brenner RJ, Sickles EA. Analysis of 172 subtle findings on prior normal mammograms in women with breast cancer detected at follow-up screening. Radiology 2003;226:494–503
16. Sickles EA. Successful methods to reduce false-positive mammography interpretations. Radiol Clin North Am 2000;38:693–700
17. Rosen EL, Baker JA, Soo MS. Malignant lesions initially subjected to short-term mammographic follow-up. Radiology 2002;223: 221–228
18. Samardar P, de Paredes ES, Grimes MM, Wilson JD. Focal asymmetric densities seen at mammography: US and pathologic correlation. Radiographics 2002;22:19–33

■ Case 7–1

Special Features   Asymmetry

Clinical History   A 38-year-old woman presents for screening.

Physical Examination   Normal exam

Radiologic Findings

Mammography

Figure 7–3 Mediolateral oblique (MLO) and craniocaudal (CC) views. **(A)** Right MLO, **(B)** right CC, **(C)** right MLO spot compression, and **(D)** right CC spot compression views. There is an ill-defined oval focal asymmetry (*square*) in the inferior inner breast.

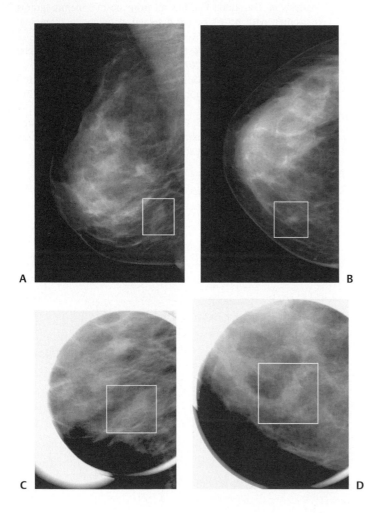

Ultrasonography

Figure 7–3 (E) Right breast sonogram. The mammographic asymmetry corresponds to an oval solid hypoechoic mass.

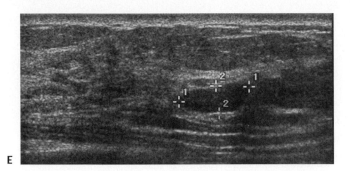

E

Management   BI-RADS category 4, suspicious. Biopsy should be considered.

Pathologic Diagnosis

Benign

Fibroadenoma

Pearls and Pitfalls

- On the basis of the sonogram, this mass may be assessed as probably benign (category 3). However, the poorly defined mammographic margins contributed to assessing this lesion as a category 4A.

■ Case 7–2

Special Features   Asymmetry

Clinical History   A 48-year-old woman presents for screening.

Physical Examination   Normal exam

Radiologic Findings

Mammography

Figure 7–4 Mediolateral oblique (MLO) and craniocaudal (CC) views. **(A)** Left MLO and **(B)** left CC mammograms. In the MLO view, there is a focal asymmetry with architectural distortion (*square*). The biopsy clip marks the location of this lesion in both views.

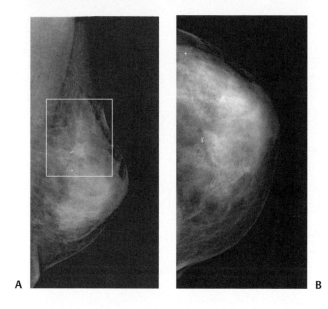

A   B

Magnetic Resonance Imaging

Figure 7–4 (C) Bilateral breast MRI (subtraction series: 2 minutes after injection of contrast). Initial ultrasound examination is negative, so an MRI is performed. In the left breast, there is a small enhancing lesion in the 12 o'clock position that corresponds to the mammographic asymmetry.

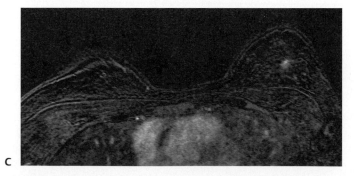

C

Ultrasonography

Figure 7–4 (D) Left breast sonogram. After magnetic resonance imaging (MRI), the sonographic exam identified a spiculated solid mass that corresponds to both the MRI and the mammogram.

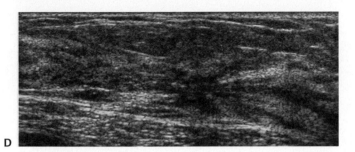

D

Management   BI-RADS category 4, suspicious. Biopsy should be considered.

Pathologic Diagnosis

Benign

Radial sclerosing lesion (radial scar)

Pearls and Pitfalls

- Radial scars are a diagnostic challenge because they commonly present as architectural distortions with or without focal asymmetry in only one view. The reason these lesions are commonly identified in only one position mammographically is that they are similar to surgical scars in shape: in one plane, they are broad, but in the orthogonal plane, they are extremely thin. This planar shape is also generally evident sonographically.

■ Case 7–3

Special Features   Asymmetry

Clinical History   An 82-year-old woman presents for screening.

Physical Examination   Normal exam

Radiologic Findings

Mammography

Figure 7–5 Mediolateral oblique (MLO) and craniocaudal (CC) views. **(A)** Left MLO mammogram. **(B)** Left CC mammogram 1 year prior. **(C)** Left MLO mammogram. **(D)** Left CC mammogram, current exam. Since the previous year (**A** and **B**), an asymmetry has developed in the upper inner quadrant.

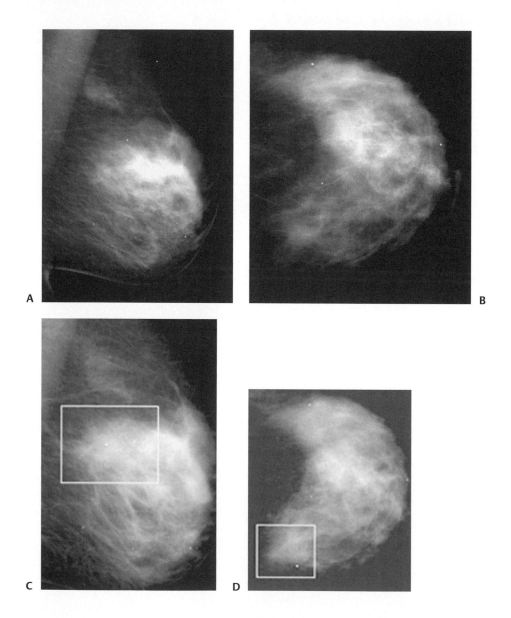

Mammography (continued)

Figure 7–5 (**E**) Left MLO spot compression mammogram. (**F**) Left CC spot compression mammogram. Spot compression views did not clarify the margins of this asymmetry.

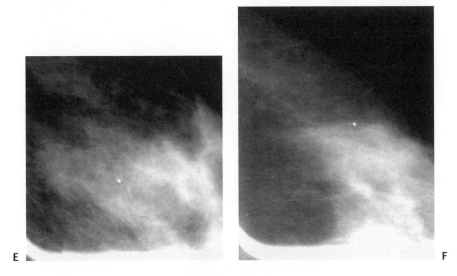

E   F

Ultrasonography

Figure 7–5 (**G**) Left breast sonogram. In the 10:30 position, the mammographic asymmetry corresponds to an irregular hypoechoic solid mass.

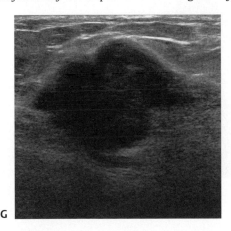

G

Management   BI-RADS category 4, suspicious. Biopsy should be considered.

Pathologic Diagnosis

Malignant

Infiltrating ductal carcinoma

Pearls and Pitfalls

- New asymmetries were previously described as neodensities or developing densities: areas in which the tissues are increasingly radiopaque, but the focus or region cannot be characterized as a mass. When the asymmetry is localized in multiple views, sonography is a useful method to further characterize and assess the asymmetry.

■ Case 7–4

Special Features Asymmetry

Clinical History A 68-year-old woman presents for screening.

Physical Examination Normal exam

Radiologic Findings

Mammography

Figure 7–6 Mediolateral (ML), mediolateral oblique (MLO), and craniocaudal (CC) views. **(A)** Left MLO, **(B)** left CC, **(C)** left ML, **(D)** left MLO spot compression, and **(E)** left CC spot compression mammograms. In the CC view, there is a central oval asymmetry with spiculations. This asymmetry is not well identified on the MLO view. In retrospect, the lesion is at 6 o'clock (marked by a square on MLO, ML, and MLO spot compression views), so the MLO spot compression views are too high and do not localize the lesion.

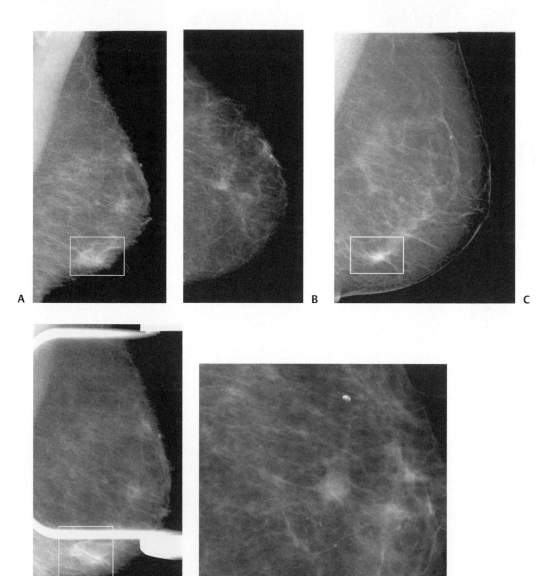

A B C

D E

Ultrasonography

Figure 7–6 (F) Left breast sonogram. At the 6 o'clock position, there is an irregular hypoechoic solid mass that corresponds to the mammographic asymmetry.

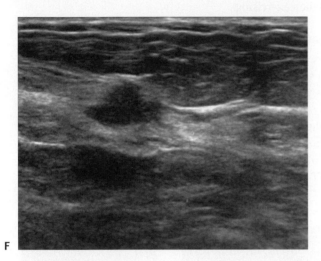

F

Management   BI-RADS category 4, suspicious. Biopsy should be considered.

Pathologic Diagnosis

Malignant

Infiltrating ductal carcinoma

Pearls and Pitfalls

- This case illustrates a disadvantage of spot compression views. With asymmetries, this technique may fail because the operator may not have reliable landmarks to localize the lesion in two views.

■ Case 7–5

Special Features   Asymmetry

Clinical History   A 29-year-old woman noticed a left breast lump when exercising.

Physical Examination   Left breast: Lump at the 6 o'clock position.

Radiologic Findings

Mammography

Figure 7–7 Mediolateral oblique (MLO) and craniocaudal (CC) views. **(A)** Right MLO, **(B)** left MLO, **(C)** right CC, and **(D)** left CC mammograms. Radiopaque marker denotes location of palpable lump. There is a focal asymmetry in the 6 o'clock position (*square*). On the screening images, the margins are only visible on the CC view.

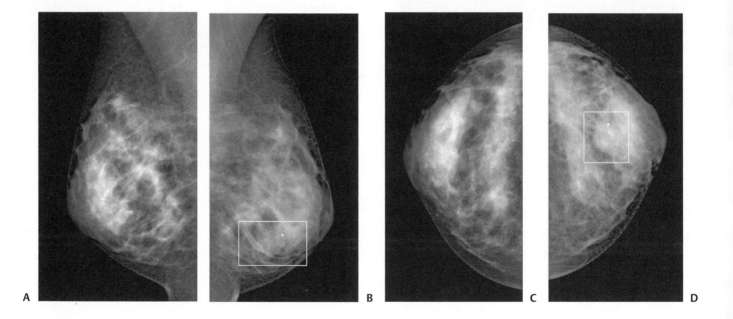

A   B   C   D

Ultrasonography

Figure 7–7 (E) Left breast sonogram. The palpable asymmetry at 6 o'clock corresponds to a hypoechoic oval solid mass with mildly indistinct margins.

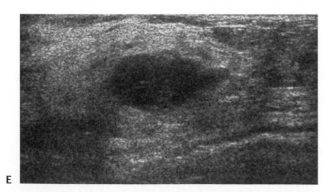

E

Magnetic Resonance Imaging

Figure 7–7 (F) Bilateral breast MRI (subtraction series: 2 minutes after injection of contrast). Left breast has an oval, rapidly enhancing mass at 6 o'clock that corresponds to the sonographic mass. No other masses or suspicious adenopathy are identified.

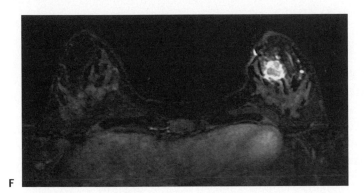

F

Management BI-RADS category 4, suspicious. Biopsy should be considered.

Pathologic Diagnosis

Malignant

Infiltrating ductal carcinoma

Pearls and Pitfalls

- Even with digital mammography, large masses may be obscured by surrounding parenchyma and present as subtle asymmetries. When asymmetries are palpable, they can be easily assessed sonographically.

■ Case 7–6

Special Features   Asymmetry

Clinical History   A 48-year-old woman presents for screening.

Physical Examination   Normal exam

Radiologic Findings

Mammography

Figure 7–8 Mediolateral oblique (MLO) and craniocaudal (CC) views. **(A)** Right MLO, **(B)** left MLO, **(C)** right CC, and **(D)** left CC mammogram. At the left 9 o'clock position, there is a vague asymmetry (*square*). **(E)** Left MLO spot magnification compression and **(F)** left CC spot magnification compression mammograms. The asymmetry is visible on the CC spot magnification view only. However, both magnification views demonstrate periareolar heterogeneous calcifications.

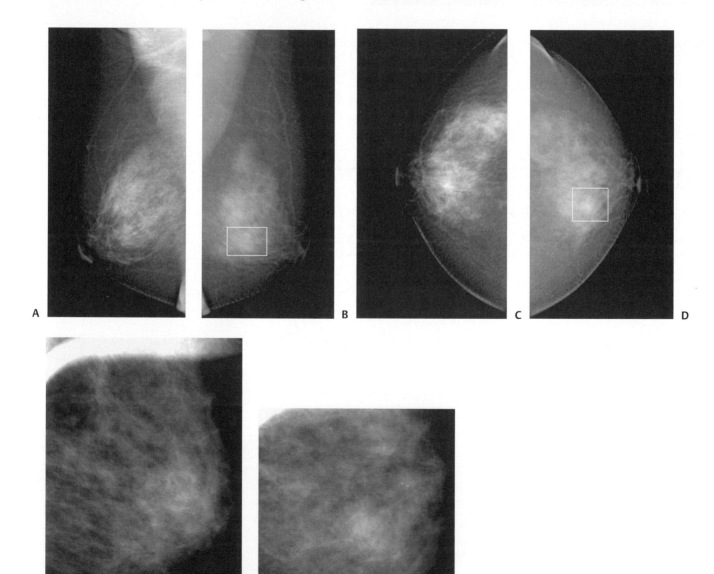

Ultrasonography

Figure 7–8 (G) At the 9 o'clock position, there is a mass (M) associated with abnormally dilated ducts (d) that extend to the nipple (N). The ducts are filled with calcifications and soft tissue material.

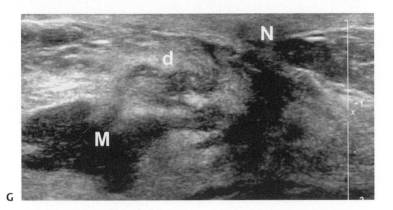

G

Magnetic Resonance Imaging

Figure 7–8 (H) Bilateral breast MRI (subtraction series: 2 minutes after injection of contrast). Left breast has an enhancing mass at 9 o'clock associated with abnormally enhancing ducts that extend to the nipple.

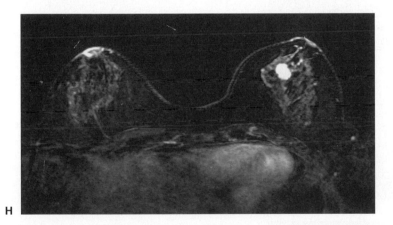

H

Management   BI-RADS category 4, suspicious. Biopsy should be considered.

Pathologic Diagnosis

Malignant

Infiltrating ductal carcinoma

Comments on Histology   There was associated high-grade ductal carcinoma in situ (DCIS).

Pearls and Pitfalls

- Although asymmetries commonly represent an overlap of benign parenchyma, whenever indirect signs of malignancy are identified on additional diagnostic views, including microcalcifications, architectural distortion, skin thickening, or nipple inversion, aggressive characterization, including sonography, should be performed.

■ Case 7–7

Special Features   Asymmetry

Clinical History   A 59-year-old woman presents who had excision of left atypical ductal hyperplasia 9 years ago.

Physical Examination   Normal exam; well-healed left breast scar.

Radiologic Findings

Mammography

Figure 7–9 Mediolateral oblique (MLO) and craniocaudal (CC) views. **(A)** Left MLO and **(B)** left CC mammograms performed 1 year prior to current exam. **(C)** Left MLO and **(D)** left CC mammograms (current screening exam). Linear marker denotes excisional scar. Since last year, there has been development of an oval asymmetry (*square*) associated with the scar visible only on the CC view.

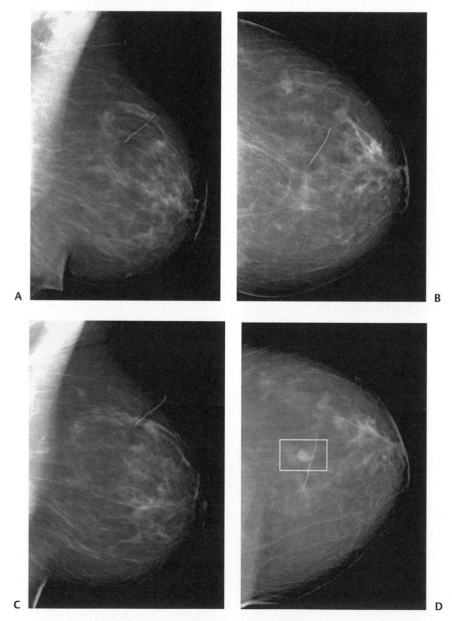

Ultrasonography

Figure 7–9 (E) Left breast sonogram. The mammographic asymmetry adjacent to the scar is an irregular hypoechoic solid mass.

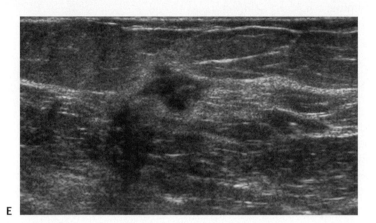

E

Management   BI-RADS category 4, suspicious. Biopsy should be considered.

Pathologic Diagnosis

Malignant

Infiltrating ductal carcinoma

Pearls and Pitfalls

- Women with atypical ductal hyperplasia have 4–5 times the risk of the general population for developing breast cancer. Therefore, new asymmetries in these women should be evaluated aggressively.[5]

■ Case 7–8

Special Features   Asymmetry

Clinical History   A 63-year-old woman presents for screening.

Physical Examination   Normal exam

Radiologic Findings

Mammography

Figure 7–10 Mediolateral oblique (MLO) and craniocaudal (CC) views. **(A)** Right MLO, **(B)** left MLO, **(C)** right CC, and **(D)** left CC mammograms. In the right MLO view, there is an oval asymmetry. **(E)** Right MLO spot compression and **(F)** right CC spot compression views. Even with spot compression, the asymmetry is difficult to identify.

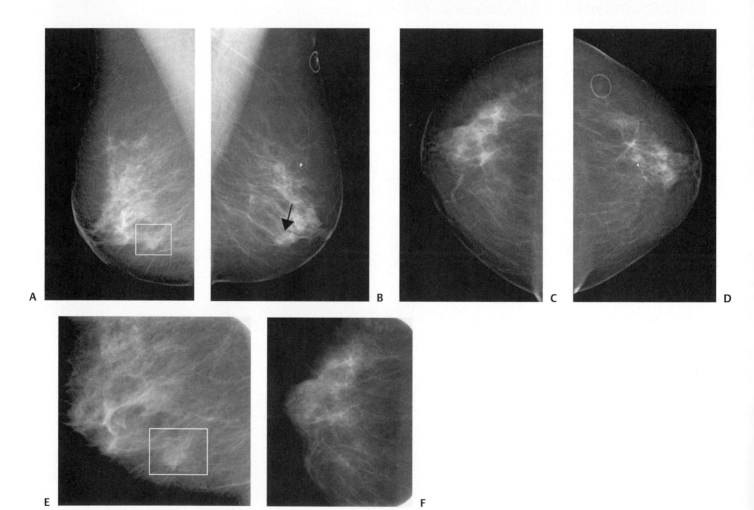

Ultrasonography

Figure 7–10 (G) Right breast sonogram. The mammographic asymmetry corresponds to an irregular hypoechoic solid mass at the 6 o'clock position.

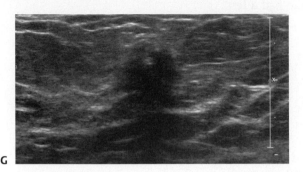

G

Management   BI-RADS category 4, suspicious. Biopsy should be considered.

Pathologic Diagnosis

Malignant

Invasive lobular carcinoma

Pearls and Pitfalls

- Lobular carcinoma commonly presents as an asymmetry probably because of its diffusely infiltrative spread. Other mammographic presentations include architectural distortion and spiculated mass. Calcifications occur in only ~20% of these malignancies.

■ Case 7–9

Special Features   Asymmetry

Clinical History   A 72-year-old woman presents for screening. She had a left lumpectomy for cancer 11 years ago.

Physical Examination   Left breast: Normal healed lumpectomy scar at the 12 o'clock position.

Radiologic Findings

Mammography

Figure 7–11 Mediolateral (ML) and craniocaudal (CC) views. **(A)** Left ML and **(B)** left CC mammograms. In the inner medial breast, there is an ill-defined asymmetry (*square*).

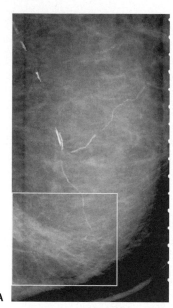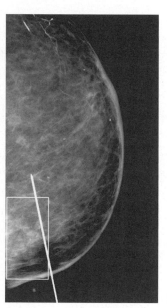

A   B

Management   BI-RADS category 4, suspicious. Biopsy should be considered.

Pathologic Diagnosis

Malignant

Invasive lobular carcinoma

Pearls and Pitfalls

- When the cells of invasive lobular carcinoma spread loosely through fat, the resulting mammographic mass commonly is not very dense, and the mass may appear to contain islands of fat, as shown in this example.

■ Case 7–10

Special Features   Asymmetry

Clinical History   An 80-year-old woman presents for screening.

Physical Examination   Right breast: Mildly diffusely firmer than left without a focal mass.

Radiologic Findings

Mammography

Figure 7–12 Mediolateral oblique (MLO) and craniocaudal (CC) views. **(A)** Right MLO, **(B)** left MLO, **(C)** right CC, and **(D)** left CC mammograms. The right breast exhibits global asymmetry associated with periareolar skin thickening and nipple inversion. **(E)** Right MLO spot compression and **(F)** right CC spot compression mammograms. Compression views confirm the diffuse asymmetry.

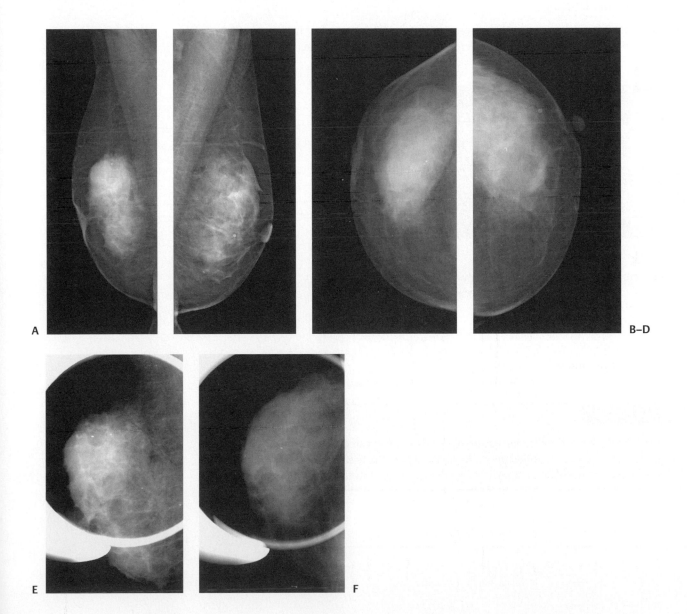

A   B–D

E   F

Ultrasonography

Figure 7–12 (G) Right breast sonogram. Wide field of view sonography demonstrates that an irregular hypoechoic mass has replaced most of the patient's glandular tissue.

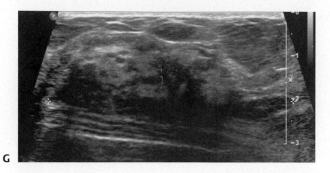

G

Magnetic Resonance Imaging

Figure 7–12 (H) Bilateral breast MRI (subtraction series: 2 minutes after injection of contrast). There is diffuse rapid enhancement of right glandular tissue.

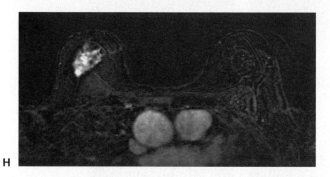

H

Management   BI-RADS category 5, highly suggestive of malignancy

Pathologic Diagnosis

Malignant

Invasive lobular carcinoma

Pearls and Pitfalls

- As a result of the diffuse infiltrative nature of invasive lobular carcinoma, this neoplasm is sometimes not identified until it involves most of the breast, producing a diffusing dense breast that is generally smaller than the contralateral breast.

■ Case 7–11

Special Features   Asymmetry

Clinical History   A 46-year-old woman presents with right breast thickening.

Physical Examination   Right breast: Large area of thickening or firmness in the upper outer quadrant.

Radiologic Findings

Mammography

Figure 7–13 Mediolateral oblique (MLO) and craniocaudal (CC) views. **(A)** Right MLO, **(B)** left MLO, **(C)** right CC, and **(D)** left CC mammograms. The right breast exhibits global asymmetry compared with the left breast. **(E)** Right MLO spot magnification and **(F)** right CC spot magnification mammograms. Associated with the asymmetry is a cluster of fine pleomorphic calcifications in the upper outer quadrant.

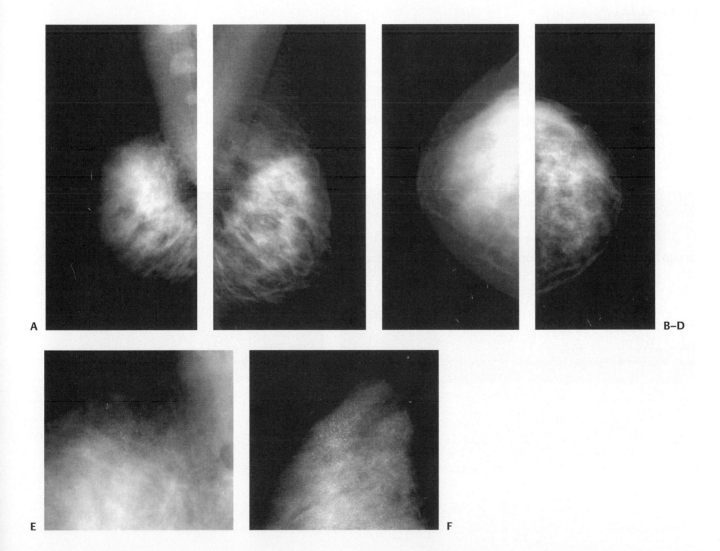

A   B–D

E   F

Ultrasonography

Figure 7–13 (G) Right breast sonogram. In the upper outer quadrant, there is an irregular hypoechoic mass with calcifications. This mass corresponds to the mammographic cluster of calcifications.

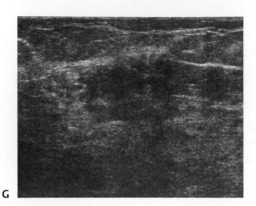

G

Magnetic Resonance Imaging

Figure 7–13 (H) Bilateral breast MRI (subtraction series: 2 minutes after injection of contrast). There is extensive rapid contrast enhancement of the right breast. On other images, there is also abnormal enhancement of enlarged right axillary nodes. **(I)** Computed tomography–positron emission tomography (CT-PET) scan. There is abnormal uptake in the right breast. This study confirmed the abnormal right axillary adenopathy and also found abnormal supraclavicular adenopathy. Furthermore, there were multiple focal bony metastases identified in the ribs (*arrow*). Sternal metastastis were evident on other images.

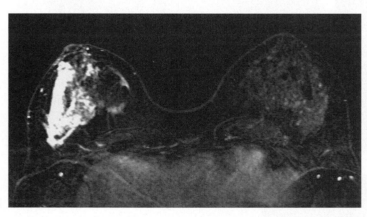

H

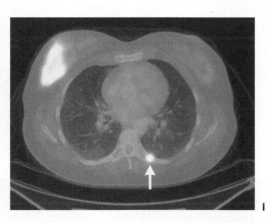

I

Management   BI-RADS category 5, highly suggestive of malignancy

Pathologic Diagnosis

Malignant

Infiltrating ductal carcinoma

Pearls and Pitfalls

- Global asymmetry may be due to benign asymmetric breast tissue or to an infiltrative mass. Global asymmetry is suspicious when there is any associated architectural distortion (e.g., trabecular thickening), microcalcifications, lymphadenopathy, skin thickening, skin retraction, or nipple inversion.

8 Digital Mammographic Characteristics of Architectural Distortion

Like asymmetries, there are few studies comparing the appearance of architectural distortion on digital mammography to screen-film mammography. Clinical investigators report small numbers of cases with either very few[1] or moderate[2] discrepancies in assessment between the two techniques for this finding. However, in these studies, the overall difference in cancer detection is not significant, and no unique cause for these discrepancies is reported.

■ General Evaluation of Architectural Distortion

To identify architectural distortion, it is important to understand the appearance of normal breast architecture. Normally, the edges of the fibroglandular tissue consist of curvilinear lines that are oriented toward the nipple. This radiating linear pattern is disrupted only by blood vessels. Adjacent to the subcutaneous fat, Cooper's ligaments form a scalloped edge. The fibroglandular edges of the breast gradually decrease in density toward the chest wall and axilla. In patients with scattered or heterogeneously dense fibroglandular composition, the edges form ill-defined curvilinear feathery borders. In patients with extremely dense composition, the edges adjacent to the axilla and chest wall commonly have the same scalloped appearance as the anterior subcutaneous parenchymal border. These patients generally exhibit a curvilinear or rounded superior border on the mediolateral oblique (MLO) view and the medial and lateral corners of the craniocaudal (CC) view.

Architectural distortion consists of straight lines, lines not oriented toward the nipple, and angular edges. It may be divided into three main locations: peripheral, central, and subareolar. Peripheral architectural distortion is readily visible in all categories of breast composition. This type of distortion is due to a lesion projecting beyond the normal fibroglandular edge or is the result of a lesion producing fibrosis or spiculation in the periphery of the fibroglandular tissue. A mass projecting beyond the fibroglandular edge is generally easy to detect: there is a focal convex margin. However, identification may be difficult if the mass is small (<5 mm) and extends outside the field of view of the mammogram. In this case, one must spot the thin "trail" of abnormal tissue that commonly connects the mass to the main fibroglandular density.

When a peripheral mass causes retraction of surrounding tissues in the posterior one third of the breast near the chest wall, the glandular tissue forms a horizontal V, which has been labeled the "tent sign." When distortion occurs in the superior fibroglandular border, the edge of the tissue becomes pointed, like an arrowhead. Furthermore, the density of this "arrow" is often slightly higher than the opposite side. This superior distortion is subtle; so long-term comparison examinations are useful to demonstrate the progression of distortion. If the superior fibroglandular edge is triangular, asymmetric with the opposite side, and has changed over time, one should be suspicious of a mass.

Architectural distortion in the central portion of the fibroglandular tissue is a lesion that consists of the intersection of multiple straight lines resembling the intersecting spokes of a wagon wheel. These lines are not directed to the nipple. There may be associated trabecular thickening or focal asymmetry. Central architectural distortion is challenging or impossible to identify in patients with heterogeneously dense or extremely dense breasts because the lesion is obscured by the surrounding breast parenchyma. Architectural distortion is even problematic to identify in breast with scattered fibroglandular composition, particularly if the breast has numerous ropy lines.

The final location of architectural distortion is the subareolar region. This is a complicated area in which to spot lesions, as there are generally many linear structures intersecting in this area. Fortunately, this area is better identified with digital mammography. In examining the subareolar region, one should note other associated abnormalities, such as nipple inversion, skin thickening, and calcifications.

If architectural distortion is recognized, the imager should first inquire if the distortion is due to a benign scar.[3] If the distortion is a scar, then it is benign unless it has increased in size or density or has developed associated abnormalities, such as suspicious calcifications. Because neoplastic changes in architectural distortion from lumpectomy may be slow, the imager should be prepared to review several comparison examinations to determine stability (**Table 8–1**).

With digital mammography, manipulation of brightness and contrast may improve conspicuity of the distortion. However, spot compression is often necessary to exaggerate the distortion. If the distortion is small or if calcifications are present, then magnification views are useful.[4]

Sometimes the architectural distortion is visible on only one view. Furthermore, if close examination of this lesion demonstrates that the center of the abnormality is

Table 8–1   BI-RADS Assessments for Mammographic Architectural Distortion Findings

BI-RADS Assessment	Definition	Examples of Mammographic Architectural Distortion Findings
Category 1	Negative	Overlap of normal fibroglandular tissue
Category 2	Benign finding	Benign known stable surgical scar
Category 3	Probably benign finding; initial short-term interval follow-up	
Category 4	Suspicious abnormality; biopsy should be considered	Architectural distortion
Category 5	Highly suspicious of malignancy	Architectural distortion associated with highly suspicious malignant findings (architectural distortion, skin thickening, nipple inversion, trabecular thickening, skin retraction, or malignant microcalcifications)

BI-RADS, Breast Imaging Reporting and Data System.

not high density and the spiculations consist of thick dark lines alternating with thin white lines, a diagnosis of radial scar should be considered.[5,6] Because radial scars are usually difficult to pinpoint on orthogonal views, the radiologist may distinguish these abnormalities by performing either shallow oblique views or rolled views. (See Chapter 7 for these techniques.) Small differences in patient position will allow easier localization of subtle abnormalities. Localization of architectural distortion is important because this lesion is virtually always a Breast Imaging Reporting and Data System (BI-RADS) category 4 (suspicious) or category 5 (highly suspicious) finding.

The most common assessment errors associated with architectural distortion are (1) missing subtle architectural distortion, (2) assuming the architectural distortion is benign if it has not changed in 1 to 2 years, and (3) poor localization of architectural distortion. To avoid missing subtle architectural distortion, it is imperative to compare each breast region systematically to the contralateral area. This approach allows any asymmetric architecture to be selected and analyzed.

Architectural distortion changes slowly, is subtle, and may be overlooked. As a result, an obvious neoplasm can be missed if it is assumed that the architectural distortion is benign after the abnormality has been stable for 1 to 2 years.[7] When an architectural distortion does not correspond to a benign scar, the lesion should be assessed as BI-RADS category 4 (suspicious) and biopsied.

It is often difficult to localize an architectural distortion even if the finding is not due to a radial scar. If mammographic architectural distortion is present, even in only one view, the lesion should be treated seriously and aggressively localized. Sonography should not be a substitute for systematic mammographic localization. Furthermore, because mammographic architectural distortion commonly has a subtle sonographic appearance, mammographic architectural distortion should not be "downgraded" by a negative sonogram. When the mammographic architectural distortion is associated with a suspicious sonographic mass, sonographic biopsy may be performed.[8–10] However, in the absence of a sonographic mass, mammographic biopsy should be performed.

References

1. Venta LA, Hendrick RE, Adler YT. Rates and causes of disagreement in interpretation of full-field digital mammography and film-screen mammography in a diagnostic setting. Am J Roentgenol 2001;176:1241–1248
2. Lewin JM, D'Orsi CJ, Hendrick RE. Clinical comparison of full-field digital mammography and screen-film mammography for detection of breast cancer. Am J Roentgenol 2002;179:671–677
3. Sickles EA, Herzog KA. Intramammary scar tissue: a mimic of the mammographic appearance of carcinoma. Am J Roentgenol 1980;135:349–352
4. Tabar LK, Dean PB, Tot T. Mammographic-histologic correlation of tumor masses asymmetric densities, and architectural distortion. In: Feig S, ed. Breast Imaging. Oak Brook, IL: RSNA; 2005:9–29
5. Tabar LK, Dean PB. Teaching Atlas of Mammography. New York: Thieme Medical Publishers; 2001:93–96,102–106

6. Adler DD, Helvie MA, Oberman HA. Radial sclerosing lesion of the breast: mammographic features. Radiology 1990;176:737–740
7. Rosen EL, Baker JA, Soo MS. Malignant lesions initially subjected to short-term mammographic follow-up. Radiology 2002;223:221–228
8. Rosen EL, Soo MS, Bentley RC. Focal fibrosis: a common breast lesion diagnosed at imaging-guided core biopsy. Am J Roentgenol 1999;173:1657–1662
9. Venta LA, Hendrick RE, Adler YT. Rates and causes of disagreement in interpretation of full-field digital mammography and film-screen mammography in a diagnostic setting. Am J Roentgenol 2001;176:1241–1248
10. Samardar P, de Paredes ES, Grimes MM, Wilson JD. Focal asymmetric densities seen at mammography: US and pathologic correlation. Radiographics 2002;22:19–33

■ Case 8–1

Special Features   Architectural distortion

Clinical History   A 72-year-old woman who had previous benign right breast biopsy presents for screening.

Physical Examination   Right breast: Faint scar near the 12 o'clock position.

Radiologic Findings

Mammography

Figure 8–1 Mediolateral oblique (MLO) and craniocaudal views. **(A)** Right MLO, **(B)** right CC, and **(C)** right CC spot compression mammograms. In the 12 o'clock position, there is architectural distortion (noted by a square in the CC view) associated with retraction of the posterior edge of the parenchyma. The architectural distortion appears more prominent than in previous exams.

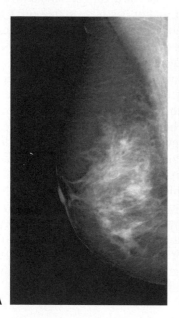
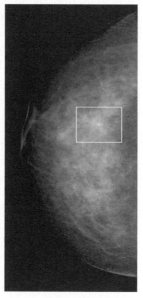
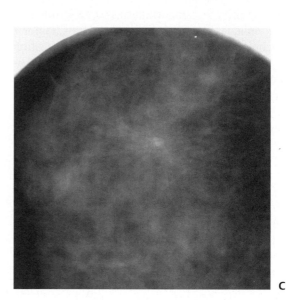

A   B   C

Management   BI-RADS category 4, suspicious. Biopsy should be considered.

Pathologic Diagnosis

Benign

Scar

Pearls and Pitfalls

- Lesions distort the posterior edge of the parenchyma in two ways: either by creating a curvilinear bulge or by retracting the edge. The retraction of the edge creates a V shape, which has been labeled the "tent sign."

■ Case 8–2

Special Features   Architectural distortion

Clinical History   A 41-year-old woman presents for screening.

Physical Examination   Normal exam

Radiologic Findings

Mammography

Figure 8–2 Mediolateral oblique (MLO) and craniocaudal (CC) views. **(A)** Right MLO, **(B)** left MLO, **(C)** right CC, **(D)** left CC, **(E)** right MLO spot compression, and **(F)** right CC spot compression mammograms. In the right 12 o'clock position, there is architectural distortion that is better identified on the MLO views (marked with a square on the MLO view).

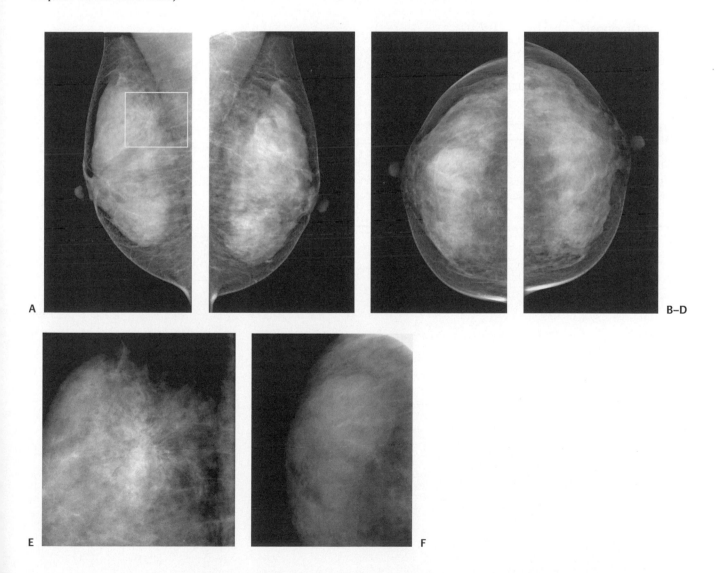

Ultrasonography

Figure 8–2 (G) Right breast sonogram. The mammographic architectural distortion corresponds to an irregular, hypoechoic solid mass.

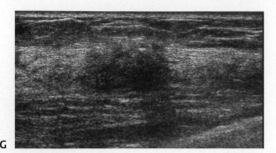

G

Management BI-RADS category 5, highly suggestive of malignancy

Pathologic Diagnosis

Benign

Radial sclerosing lesion (radial scar)

Pearls and Pitfalls

- Lesions with architectural distortion are some of the most suspicious abnormalities in the breast. Unless the distortion is due to a benign scar, a spiculated lesion, even when visible in only one view, is highly suspicious when it corresponds to an abnormal sonographic mass.

■ Case 8–3

Special Features   Architectural distortion

Clinical History   A 34-year-old woman has difficulty breast-feeding her baby from the right breast.

Physical Examination   Right breast: Subareolar lump present. Left breast: Normal exam.

Radiologic Findings

Mammography

Figure 8–3 Mediolateral oblique (MLO) and craniocaudal (CC) views. **(A)** Right MLO, **(B)** left MLO, **(C)** right CC, and **(D)** left CC mammograms. **(E)** Enlargement of C. There is skin thickening and trabecular coarsening (*arrows in* **E**) in the right periareolar and subareolar area.

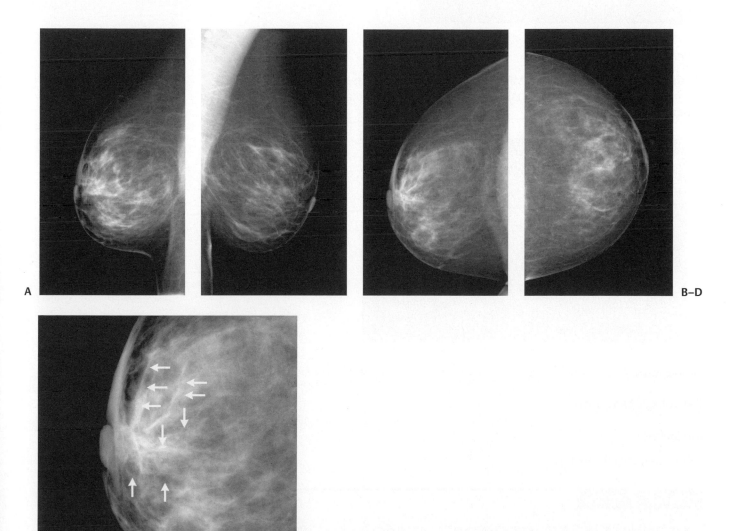

A

B–D

E

Ultrasonography

Figure 8–3 (F) Right breast sonogram. Under the nipple (N), there is a solid, hypoechoic, heavily shadowing mass. Skin thickening (*arrows*) is also apparent.

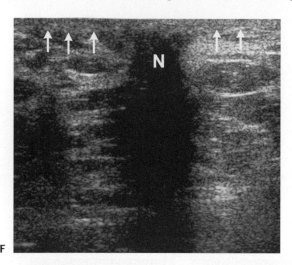

F

Magnetic Resonance Imaging

Figure 8–3 (G) Bilateral breast MRI (subtraction series: 2 minutes after injection of contrast). There is an abnormally enhancing right subareolar mass extending into the nipple.

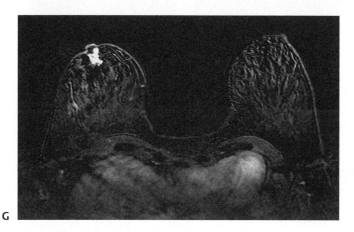

G

Management   BI-RADS category 4, suspicious. Biopsy should be considered.

Pathologic Diagnosis

Malignant

Infiltrating ductal carcinoma

Pearls and Pitfalls

- About 1 in 3000 to 10,000 pregnancies will be complicated by breast cancer. The most common symptoms are a palpable lump or bloody nipple discharge. Studies have found that more than three quarters of all pregnant patients with breast cancer have mammographic abnormalities. The most common histology of these patients is infiltrating ductal carcinoma.

■ Case 8–4

Special Features   Architectural distortion

Clinical History   A 90-year-old woman notes new nipple inversion.

Physical Examination   Right breast: Nipple inversion associated with subareolar firmness. Left breast: Normal exam.

Radiologic Findings

Mammography

Figure 8–4 Mediolateral oblique (MLO) and craniocaudal (CC) views. **(A)** Right MLO, **(B)** left MLO, **(C)** right CC, and **(D)** left CC mammograms. **(E)** Enlargement of **(A)** There is a right subareolar spiculated mass (M) with periareolar skin thickening and spiculations (*arrows*).

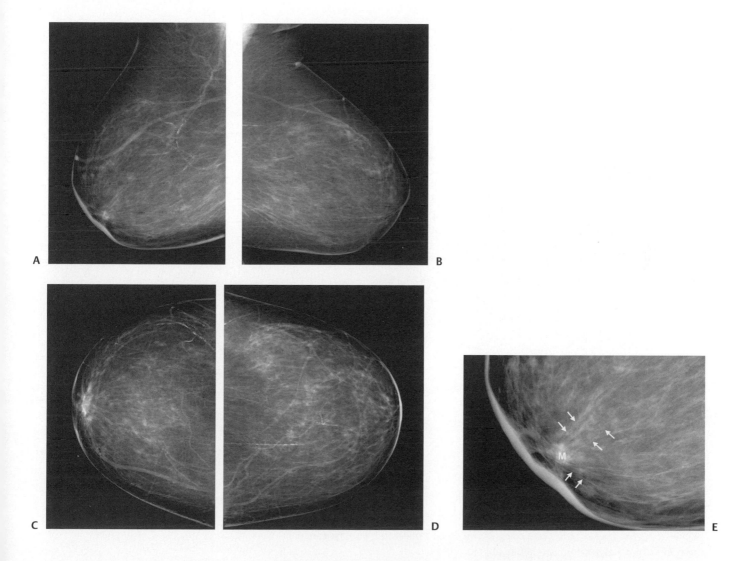

Ultrasonography

Figure 8–4 (F) Right breast sonogram. The subareolar mass corresponds to an isoechoic mass (M), which produces an abrupt ductal (D) obstruction. Spiculations (*arrows*) extend from the mass, as in the mammogram. Skin thickening (S) is also present.

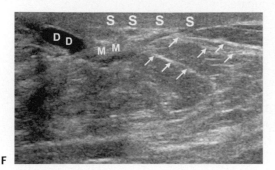

Management   BI-RADS category 5, highly suggestive of malignancy

Pathologic Diagnosis

Malignant

Invasive ductal carcinoma

Pearls and Pitfalls

- Subareolar architectural distortion is difficult to identify because there are many normal anatomic lines that converge under the nipple. However, with the nipple in profile, these lines should gradually converge to a point under the nipple. In this case, the lines intersect but do not form a point; instead, they form a cross (**Fig. 8–4A,B**).

■ Case 8–5

Special Features   Architectural distortion

Clinical History   A 64-year-old woman presents with right breast skin dimpling.

Physical Examination   Right breast: There is subtle skin dimpling in the inframammary fold at the 5 o'clock position. Left breast: Normal.

Radiologic Findings

Mammography

Figure 8–5   Mediolateral (ML) and craniocaudal (CC) views. **(A)** Right ML and **(B)** right CC mammograms. **(C)** Enlarged view of **(A)** On the ML view, there is skin thickening (S) and retraction (*arrow*) associated with an irregular mass (M).

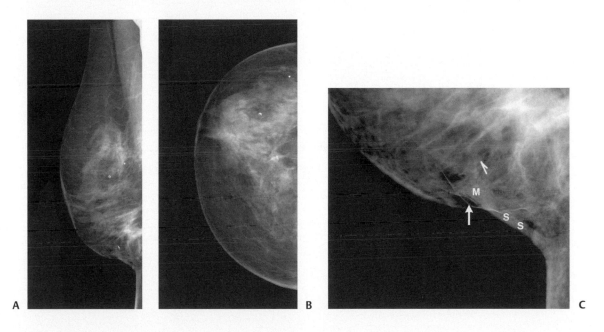

A   B   C

Ultrasonography

Figure 8–5 (D) Right breast sonogram. The mammographic findings correspond to a small hypoechoic irregular solid mass (M) with shadowing (*arrows*). Skin thickening (S) is also evident.

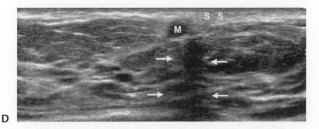

D

Management   BI-RADS category 4, suspicious. Biopsy should be considered.

Pathologic Diagnosis

Malignant

Infiltrating ductal carcinoma

Comments on Histology   3-mm infiltrating ductal carcinoma resected

Pearls and Pitfalls

- The inframammary fold or crease is a difficult area to image and evaluate. Digital manipulation of window level and width is particularly useful when trying to evaluate the extreme peripheral locations of the breast.

■ Case 8–6

Special Features   Architectural distortion

Clinical History   A 71-year-old woman presents for screening.

Physical Examination   Normal exam

Radiologic Findings

Mammography

Figure 8–6 Mediolateral oblique (MLO) and craniocaudal (CC) views. **(A)** Right MLO, **(B)** left MLO, **(C)** right CC, and **(D)** left CC mammograms. At screening, there is left architectural distortion in the central retroareolar plane on the CC view (*square*). **(E)** Left MLO labeled mammogram. **(F)** Left MLO spot compression mammogram. **(G)** Left CC spot compression mammogram. Initially, the architectural distortion is identified only on the CC view; however, after careful analysis, the spiculated mass is located on the MLO view (*square*). Besides the spiculations, there is also depression of the margin of the left superior glandular border of the breast (*arrows*). With spot compression views, the mass is visible only in the CC position.

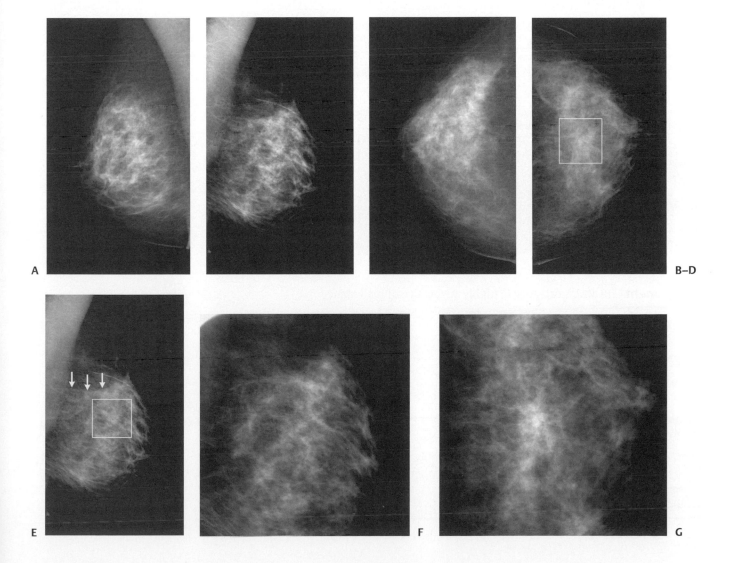

Ultrasonography

Figure 8–6 (H) Left breast sonogram. The mammographic mass corresponds to an irregular hypoechoic solid mass with heavy shadowing.

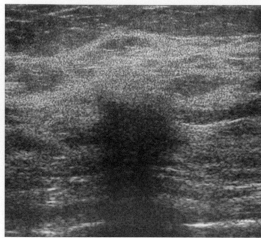

H

Magnetic Resonance Imaging

Figure 8–6 (I) Bilateral breast MRI. This sequence is performed several minutes after contrast injection, so there is normal diffuse right glandular enhancement. This image illustrates the central position of the left breast mass (*marked by a square*) that closely corresponds to the CC mammographic view.

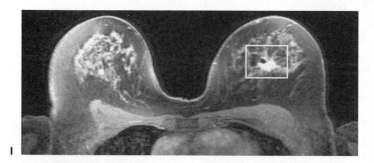

I

Management   BI-RADS category 5, highly suggestive of malignancy

Pathologic Diagnosis

Malignant

Infiltrating ductal carcinoma

Pearls and Pitfalls

- Masses located centrally may be difficult to identify when surrounded by parenchyma. This case illustrates that spot compression views may not always localize a lesion. Therefore, if the abnormality is suspicious, the imager should aggressively apply other methods to locate the lesion.

■ Case 8–7

Special Features   Architectural distortion

Clinical History   A 61-year-old woman presents with a left palpable mass.

Physical Examination   Left breast: Lump in the upper outer quadrant.

Radiologic Findings

Mammography

Figure 8–7 Mediolateral oblique (MLO) and craniocaudal (CC) views. **(A)** Left MLO, **(B)** left CC, **(C)** left MLO spot compression, and **(D)** left CC spot compression mammograms. There is an irregular mass in the upper outer quadrant. The central architecture of the breast is distorted by the straight spiculations extending from the mass into the normal parenchyma.

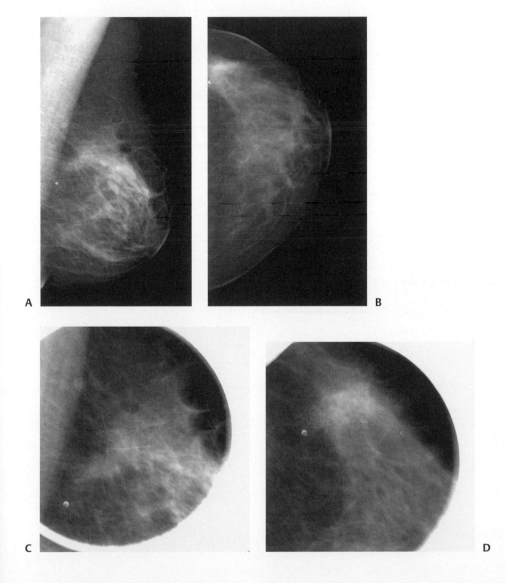

A

B

C

D

Ultrasonography

Figure 8–7 (E) Left breast sonogram. The mammographic mass corresponds to an irregular, hypoechoic, shadowing solid mass. The mass infiltrates the surrounding normal glandular tissues (*arrowheads*), thickening Cooper's ligaments (*arrows*).

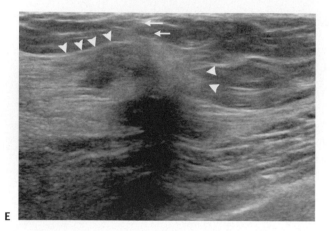

E

Management   BI-RADS category 5, highly suggestive of malignancy

Pathologic Diagnosis

Malignant

Infiltrating ductal carcinoma

Pearls and Pitfalls

- Generally, infiltrating ductal carcinoma has two main appearances on gross pathology: the stellate/scirrhous tumor and the nodular/circumscribed mass. The former type probably produces more mammographic architectural distortion than the latter. This stellate type is associated with extensive fibrosis and accounts for about two thirds of all infiltrating ductal cancers.

■ Case 8–8

Special Features Architectural distortion

Clinical History A 68-year-old woman is 3 years post–right lumpectomy.

Physical Examination Right breast: Normal lumpectomy scar. Left breast: Normal exam.

Radiologic Findings

Mammography

Figure 8–8 Mediolateral oblique (MLO) and exaggerated craniocaudal (XCCL) views. **(A)** Right MLO and **(B)** right XCCL mammograms. In the axillary tail of the breast, there is new architectural distortion (*square*) associated with an old lumpectomy site.

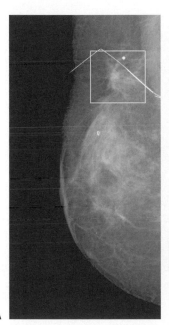
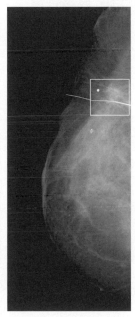

A   B

Management BI-RADS category 4, suspicious. Biopsy should be considered.

Pathologic Diagnosis

Malignant

Invasive lobular carcinoma

Pearls and Pitfalls

- The mammographic appearance of postsurgical lesions generally stabilizes ~3 to 5 years after excision. After this time, ~50% of patients still exhibit lesions, including architectural distortion, skin thickening, and other signs of parenchymal scarring. Obviously, any new or increasing architectural distortion should be aggressively evaluated.

■ Case 8–9

Special Features   Architectural distortion

Clinical History   An 80-year-old woman presents for screening.

Physical Examination   Normal exam

Radiologic Findings

Mammography

Figure 8–9 Mediolateral oblique (MLO) and craniocaudal (CC) views. **(A)** Left CC, **(B)** left 10-degree MLO, **(C)** left 20-degree MLO, and **(D)** left 45-degree (screening) MLO mammograms. In the 12 o'clock position, there is a subtle irregular mass (*square*). Coarse trabeculations or spiculations extend from the mass.

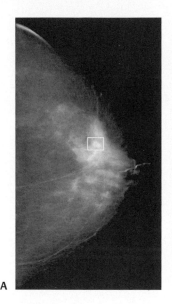
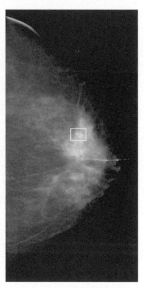
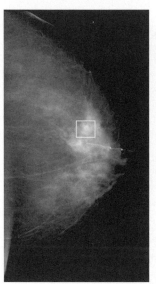
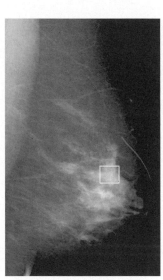

A   B   C   D

Ultrasonography

Figure 8–9 (E) Left breast sonogram. The mammographic mass corresponds to an irregular hypoechoic solid mass that shadows.

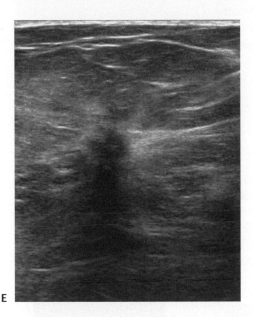

E

Management   BI-RADS category 4, suspicious. Biopsy should be considered.

Pathologic Diagnosis

Malignant

Infiltrating ductal carcinoma

Pearls and Pitfalls

- Central masses may be subtle even when associated with architectural distortion. Originally, from the screening images, the mass was thought to be closer to the 3 o'clock position, but shallow oblique views demonstrate that the mass is closer to 12:30. Identification of the location of a mass is important for determining the position of spot compression views as well as for targeting sonography for further characterization or biopsy.

■ Case 8–10

Special Features   Architectural distortion

Clinical History   A 52-year-old woman presents for a second opinion. During an outside screening evaluation, the imager identified a new area of architectural distortion on the MLO view but not on the CC view. (The area has been stable for 4 years.) The outside institution performed an ultrasound but could not identify a mass.

Physical Examination   Normal exam

Radiologic Findings

Mammography

Figure 8–10 Mediolateral oblique (MLO) and craniocaudal (CC) views. **(A)** Right MLO (57-degree screening), **(B)** right MLO (47 degrees), **(C)** right MLO (37 degrees), and **(D)** right CC mammograms. **(E)** Enlargement of architectural distortion from **(B)** Because the architectural distortion is initially not clearly identified on the CC position, shallow oblique views are produced. The architectural distortion persists in the upper breast on the shallow oblique views and corresponds to the outer breast on the CC view (architectural distortion marked with squares).

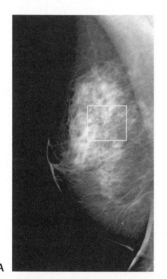 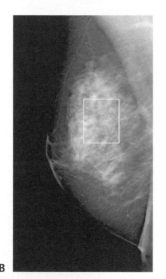 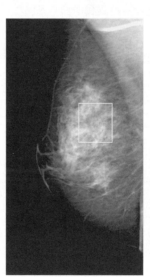 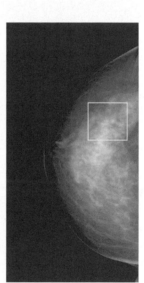

A   B   C   D

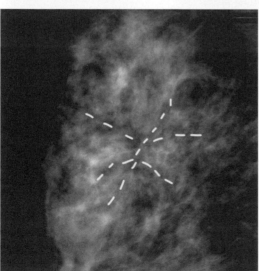

E

Ultrasonography

Figure 8–10 (F) Right breast sonogram. The architectural distortion corresponds to an irregular hypoechoic solid shadowing mass (M) with thick spiculations (*arrows*).

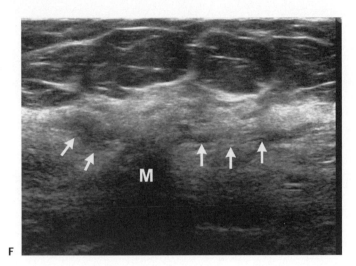

F

Management   BI-RADS category 4, suspicious. Biopsy should be considered.

Pathologic Diagnosis

Benign

Radial sclerosing lesion (radial scar)

Pearls and Pitfalls

- This case illustrates the importance of triangulating subtle architectural distortion. The shallow obliques confirm the position of the distortion in multiple views and contributes to greater success in locating the mass sonographically.

Index

Note: Page numbers followed by f and t represent figures and tables respectively.

A
Abscess, global asymmetries and, 148
Acquisition of digital images
   equipment for, 9–11, 10f–11f
   physics, 4–7, 4f–6f
ACRIN (American College of Radiology Imaging Network), 2
Adenocarcinoma, mammary, metaplastic
     carcinoma and, 123
Adenosis, sclerosing. See Sclerosing adenosis
ADH. See Atypical ductal hyperplasia
Aluminum, mammographic density and, 28
American College of Radiology Breast Imaging
     Reporting and Data System. See BI-RADS
     assessments
American College of Radiology Imaging Network, 2
Amorphous calcifications, 20–21, 21t
   atypical ductal hyperplasia and, 59f
   ductal carcinoma in situ and, 60f, 62f, 64f
   identification difficulties, 64
   malignancy rates with, 63
   visibility, 72
Anatomic lines, convergence of, 183f, 184
Antiperspirant, mammographic density and, 28
Apocrine metaplasia
   mammography findings, 110f
   ultrasonography findings, 110f, 111
Architectural distortion, 14
   assessment errors, 177
   with associated global asymmetry, 175
   evaluation, 176–177, 177t
   in infiltrating ductal carcinoma
     elderly patient with, 187f–188f, 192f–193f
     with palpable mass, 189f–190f

     postpartum, 181f–182f, 182
     with skin dimpling, 185f
   in invasive carcinoma
     ductal, 183f–184f
     lobular, 191f
   and normal breast architecture, 176
   rate of change in, 177
   scars and, 178f
     lumpectomy scar, 191f
     radial sclerosing scar, 179f–180f, 194f–195f
   subareolar, 183f, 184
   types, 176
Artifacts, 7
   screen-film vs. digital images, 14
Asymmetric densities. See also Mammographic asymmetry
   in invasive lobular carcinoma, 172
   mass localization and, 104f–105f
   neo- or developing, 159
Atherosclerosis, vascular calcifications in, 32f
Attenuation, of incident x-ray keV, 5, 5t
Atypical ductal hyperplasia
   with amorphous calcifications, 59f
   apocrine metaplasia and, 111
   breast cancer risk and, 59, 167
   DCIS vs., 56
   with fine pleomorphic calcifications, 73f, 74f–75f, 76, 76f
   malignancy rates in, 73
   with punctate calcifications, 56f
Axillary adenopathy
   in infiltrating ductal carcinoma, 137f
   in invasive ductal carcinoma, 120f–121f
Axillary lymphatic obstruction, global
     asymmetries and, 148

B

BI-RADS assessments
architectural distortion, 176–177, 177t
breast composition and, 15f–17f, 17–18, 17t
categories, 17t
mammographic asymmetries, 149, 152, 152t
evaluation methods establishing, 149, 151t
and follow-up imaging, 152
mammographic calcifications, 20–21, 21t
fine pleomorphic, in DCIS, 78, 79
masses, 91–92, 91t
shape categories, 90–91, 91t
parenchymal composition categories, 2
risk assessment in, 21
Breast anatomy
architectural distortion and, 176
BI-RADS evaluation, 15f–17f, 17–18, 17t
mammographic technique in, 14–17, 14f
Breast cancer. *See also* Ductal carcinoma; Ductal
carcinoma in situ; Infiltrating ductal carcinoma;
Invasive ductal carcinoma
atypical ductal hyperplasia and, 59, 167
axillary nodal involvement with, survival rates, 138
in pregnancy, 182
Breast density, in inflammatory carcinoma, 144
Breast Imaging Reporting and Data System. *See* BI-RADS
assessments
"Breast within the breast" appearance, hamartoma
with, 94

C

CAD. *See* Computer-aided detection
Calcifications
in benign lobules, 46f
BI-RADS assessment, 20–21, 21t
casting type, 87
coarse. *See* Coarse calcifications
detection technique, 19–20
ductal carcinoma in situ and, 20
eggshell. *See* Eggshell calcifications
evaluation approach to, 20
examination, 20
heterogeneous, in infiltrating ductal carcinoma,
164f–165f
identifying, screen-film vs. digital display, 14, 24
in lobular carcinoma, 169
popcorn. *See* Popcorn calcifications
size and morphology, 20–21, 21t
skin. *See* Skin calcifications
types, 20
vascular. *See* Vascular calcifications
Casting calcifications, 87
Cathode-ray tube displays, 11
CC views. *See* Craniocaudal views
CCDs (charge-coupled devices), in slot scanning
detector, 9–10

Central masses, identification of
subtleties in, 193
with surrounding parenchyma, 188
Cesium iodide phosphor detector system, 9, 10f
flat-panel, 9, 10f
slot scanning, 9–10
Charge-coupled devices, in slot scanning
detector, 9–10
Circumscribed masses
apocrine metaplasia, 110f
cysts, 100f, 101, 102f
with asymmetric density, 104f–105f
as solid mass sonographically, 106f, 107
with thin septation, 108f–109f
fibroadenoma, 112f, 114f
foreign bodies, 99, 99f
hamartoma, 94f
intracystic papillary carcinoma, 126f–127f
invasive ductal carcinoma, 118f, 120f–121f
invasive papillary carcinoma, 124f, 141f
lymph node, 95f
metaplastic carcinoma, 122f–123f
oil cyst, 97f–98f
pseudoangiomatous stromal hyperplasia, 116f, 117
Coarse calcifications
in fibroadenoma, 33f
dystrophic, 34f, 35f
heterogeneous. *See* Heterogeneous calcifications, coarse
lumpectomy scar with
mammography findings, 39f, 65f
ultrasonography findings, 40f
Compression, of focal asymmetry, 149
Computed radiology system, for image acquisition, 9,
10, 11f
advantages and disadvantages, 10
display specifications, 11
Computer-aided detection
screening exams and, 19–20
sensitivities, masses vs. microcalcifications, 90
CR system. *See* Computed radiology system
Craniocaudal views
architectural distortion, 176
focal asymmetries, 149, 150f, 151f, 151t
screen-film vs. digital, in screening exam, 15
CRT (cathode-ray tube) displays, 11
CsI phosphor detector system. *See* Cesium iodide
phosphor detector system
"Cut sausage" appearance, hamartoma with, 94
Cysts. *See also* Microcysts
asymmetric density and, 104f–105f
mammography findings, 100f, 101, 102f, 104f,
106f, 108f
ultrasonography findings, 100f, 102, 102f, 105f
identification accuracy, 103
as solid mass, 106f, 107
with thin septation, 109f

D
DCIS. *See* Ductal carcinoma in situ
Dead pixels, 7
del (detector element), 6
Deodorant, mammographic density and, 28
DICOM (Digital Imaging and Communications in
    Medicine)
  for image retrieval, 11
  for image storage, 11
Digital detector
  characteristic curve, screen-film vs., 4–5, 5f
  dynamic range adequacy example, 5, 5t
  modulation transfer function and, 6, 6f
  noise in, 6–7
  spatial resolution, 6, 6f
Digital image
  display. *See* Digital image display
  inversion of white-and-black presentation
      mode, 75
  pixel matrix, 4, 4f
  scaling, 11–12
  size requirements, 12, 12t
  storage. *See* Digital image storage
Digital image acquisition
  equipment for, 9–11, 10f–11f
  physics, 4–7, 4f–6f
Digital image acquisition systems
  common features, 10–11
  image packaging and, 11
Digital image display, 7
  hard copy vs. soft copy, 19
  specifications, 11–12
  system functionality, 11
Digital image storage, 7, 12–13, 12f, 12t
  DICOM and, 11, 12, 12t
  PACS and, 12–13
  requirements, 12, 12t
Digital latitude, 5
Digital Mammographic Imaging Screening
    Trial, 2
Digital mammography
  architectural distortion, 176–177, 177t
    case examples, 178–195
  asymmetries, 148–152, 150f–151f, 151t–152t
    case examples, 154–175
  benign and malignant calcifications, 19–21, 21t
    case examples, 24–89
  breast tissue density and, 2
  equipment for, 9–13, 10f–11f, 12t
  historical review, 1–2
  masses, 90–92, 91t
    case examples, 94–147
  normal breast, 14–18, 14f–17f, 17t
  physics, 4–7, 4f–6f
  as screening tool, 1
  vs. screen-film mammography

diagnostic sensitivity, 1, 2
  in inflammatory carcinoma, 144
  in large breasts, 139
  masses, 90
  skin calcifications, 14, 24
  in younger women, 2
Digital range, 5
Digital workstations, postprocessing methods and
    hanging options on, 14–15
Digital x-ray systems, for image acquisition, 9
Display, digital images. *See* Digital image display
DMIST (Digital Mammographic Imaging Screening
    Trial), 2
Doppler sonogram
  apocrine metaplasia, 110f, 111
  simple cyst with septation, 109f
Ductal carcinoma, with architectural distortion
  infiltrating. *See* Infiltrating ductal carcinoma
  invasive, 183f–184f
Ductal carcinoma in situ
  atypical ductal hyperplasia vs., 56
  calcification patterns suggesting, 77, 82
  with calcifications, 20
    amorphous, 60f, 62f, 64f
    coarse heterogeneous, 69f
    fine linear, 87, 87f
    fine pleomorphic, 77–79, 77f–85f, 82
    punctate, 53
  infiltrating ductal carcinoma and, 165
  invasive malignancies vs., 130
  as irregular mass, 130f
  vascular calcifications vs., 31
Ductal hyperplasia, atypical. *See* Atypical ductal
    hyperplasia
Dystrophic calcifications
  in fibroadenoma, 34f, 35f
  lumpectomy scar and, 40
    mammography findings, 37f, 39f
    ultrasonography findings, 40f

E
Eggshell calcifications, 20
  in cyst, 41f
Electronic grid lines, 14, 14f
  calcification localization and, 24
Electronically marked images, 108f, 109
  usefulness, 109

F
Fat
  in BI-RADS assessment, 17, 18
  in hamartoma appearance, 94
  masses with and without, 90–91
Fat islands
  focal asymmetry and, 149
  in invasive ductal carcinoma, 170

Fat necrosis
    with coarse heterogeneous calcifications, 65f
    with dystrophic calcifications, 37f
    with round calcifications, 42, 42f, 43f
Fatty hilum, in lymph nodes, 121
FDA (Food and Drug Administration), flat-panel display
    specifications, 11
Fibroadenoma, 112f
    after menopause, 34, 113
    as circumscribed mass, 112f, 114f
    with coarse calcifications, 33f
        dystrophic, 34f
        heterogeneous, 67f
    incidence, 113
    as irregular mass, 128f, 129
    with mammographic asymmetry, 154f–155f
    mammography findings
        in circumscribed mass, 112f, 114f, 115
        in irregular mass, 128f, 129
    popcorn calcifications in, 20, 33, 33f
    ultrasonography findings
        in circumscribed mass, 112f, 114f
        in irregular mass, 128f, 129
    with vascular calcifications, 34f
Fibrocystic change, with fine pleomorphic
    calcifications, 71, 71f, 72f
Fibrocystic tissue, benign
    with coarse heterogeneous calcifications, 66f
    with punctate calcifications, 55f
Fibroglandular tissue
    architectural distortion in, 176
    BI-RADS assessment, 15f–16f, 17–18
    focal asymmetries and, 148–149
    global asymmetries and, 148
    in hamartoma appearance, 94
    incident x-ray attenuation in, 5, 5t
    in normal breast architecture, 176
Fibrosis, benign
    coarse heterogeneous calcifications and, 67
    punctate calcifications in, 54f
    stromal, fine pleomorphic calcifications and, 70f
Field of view, 19
Fine linear calcifications, 21, 21t
    branching type, 21, 21t, 87
    ductal carcinoma in situ with, 87, 87f
    infiltrating ductal carcinoma with, 88f–89f
        mammography findings, 88f
        MRI findings, 89f
        ultrasonography findings, 89f
Fine pleomorphic calcifications, 21, 21t
    atypical ductal hyperplasia with, 73f, 74f–75f,
        76, 76f
    benign microcysts with, 70f
    BI-RADS assessments, 78, 79
    characteristics, 70
    classic appearance, 82

    ductal carcinoma in situ with, 77–79, 77f–85f, 82
    fibrocystic changes with, 71, 71f, 72f
    histologic correlates, 76
    invasive ductal carcinoma with, 85f
    magnification views for, advantages of, 75
    patterns suggesting DCIS, 77, 82
    visibility, 72
Fischer SenoScan, trial tests, 1
Fixed electronic structural noise, 7
Flat fielding artifacts, 7
Flat-panel displays, FDA specifications for, 11
Flat-panel mammographic detectors
    cesium iodide, 9, 10f
    display specifications, 11–12
    selenium, 9, 10f
    vs. screen-film imaging, microcalcifications and, 19
Focal asymmetries
    compressible nature, 149
    global asymmetries vs., 148–149
    lesion localization, methods for, 149, 150f–151f
    masses appearing as, 149
Food and Drug Administration, flat-panel display
    specifications, 11
Foreign bodies, 99, 99f
FOV (field of view), 19
Full-field digital systems, 10–11

G
General Electric Senographe 2000D, trial tests, 1
Global asymmetries
    causes, 148
    vs. focal asymmetries, 148–149
    work-up, 148
Gray-scale imaging
    calcification of a cystic process, 41
    microcalcifications, 20
    monitoring with, 12

H
Halo sign
    benign cysts and, 100f, 101
    fibroadenomas and, 115
Hamartoma, 94f
    varied appearance, 94
Hanging protocol options, 14–15
Heterogeneous calcifications, coarse, 21, 21t
    benign fibrocystic tissue with, 66f
    characteristics, 66
    ductal carcinoma in situ with, 69f
    fat necrosis and, 65f
    fibroadenoma with, 67f
    papilloma with sclerosis and, 68f
    recurrence rate, 65
    visibility, 68
Heterogeneously dense breasts, in BI-RADS
    assessment, 17f, 18

Hormone replacement therapy, global asymmetries and, 148
Hyperplasia
    ductal, atypical. *See* Atypical ductal hyperplasia
    lobular, 52
    stromal, pseudoangiomatous. *See* Pseudoangiomatous stromal hyperplasia

I
IHE (Integrating the Healthcare Enterprise), 13
Image. *See* Digital image
Image acquisition. *See* Digital image acquisition
Imaging protocols, for diagnostic mammography, 16–17
Incident x-ray keV, attenuation of, 5, 5t
Indirect secondary noise, 7
Infiltrating ductal carcinoma
    with architectural distortion
        in elderly patient, 187f–188f, 192f–193f
        with palpable mass, 189f–190f
        postpartum, 181f–182f, 182
        with skin dimpling, 185f
    with fine linear calcifications, 88f–89f
        mammography findings, 88f
        ultrasonography findings, 89f
    gross pathologic appearance, 190
    with mammographic asymmetry, 160f–161f
        after prior excision of atypical ductal hyperplasia, 166f–167f
        in elderly woman, 158f–159f
        heterogeneous calcifications in, 164f–165f
        outer quadrant thickening, 173f–174f
    mammography findings, 131f, 132, 133f, 135f, 137f, 139f
    MRI findings, 134f, 138f
    ultrasonography findings, 131f, 132, 133f, 135f, 138f, 140f
Inflammatory carcinoma
    mammography findings, 143f, 144, 145f
    mastitis vs., 147
    MRI findings, 144f, 146f
    occurrence, 147
    ultrasonography findings, 143f, 146f
Inframammary fold
    imaging difficulties, 186
    skin dimpling in, 185f
Integrating the Healthcare Enterprise, 13
Intracystic papillary carcinoma
    mammography findings, 126f
    ultrasonography findings, 127f
Invasive ductal carcinoma, 118f
    with architectural distortion, 183f–184f
    contralateral malignancy rates with, 86
    with fine pleomorphic calcifications, 85f
    with mammographic asymmetry, in elderly woman, 170f
    mammography findings, 118f, 120f
    MRI findings, 121f

presentation characteristics, 119
    with punctate calcifications, 57f
        and intraductal component, 58
    ultrasonography findings, 118f, 121f
Invasive lobular carcinoma
    with architectural distortion, 191f
    with mammographic asymmetry, 168f–169f
        diffusely dense, 171f–172f
Invasive malignancies
    ductal carcinoma in situ vs., 130
    sound transmission and, 123
Invasive papillary carcinoma
    characteristics and presenting symptoms, 125
    incidence, 142
    mammography findings, 124f, 141f
    ultrasonography findings, 124f, 141f
Irregular masses
    ductal carcinoma in situ, 130f
    fibroadenoma, 128f, 129
    infiltrating ductal carcinoma, 131f, 133f–135f, 137f–140f
    inflammatory carcinoma, 143f–144f, 145f–146f

L
Latitude, digital, 5
Lesions
    with architectural distortion. *See* Architectural distortion
    asymmetric. *See* Mammographic asymmetry
    with calcification. *See* Calcifications
    noncalcified. *See* Circumscribed masses; Irregular masses; Mammographic masses
    postsurgical. *See* Postsurgical lesions
Linear calcifications
    fine, 21, 21t
        branching type, 21, 21t
    thick, 20
        characteristics, 50
        in plasma cell mastitis, 49f
Lobular carcinoma
    invasive. *See* Invasive lobular carcinoma
    mammographic presentations, 169
Lobular hyperplasia, 52
Lobules, benign
    with oval and round calcifications, 46f, 47
    with punctate calcifications, 48, 48f, 51f, 53f
Lucent center calcifications, 20
    mammography findings, 25f, 26
Lucent halo. *See* Halo sign
Lumpectomy, recurrent rate for, 65
Lumpectomy scar
    architectural distortion associated with, 191f
    dystrophic calcifications within, 40
        mammography findings, 37f, 38f, 39f
        ultrasonography findings, 40f
    heterogenous coarse calcifications within, 65f

Lymph node
    in invasive ductal carcinoma, 121, 121f
    mammography findings, 95f, 96
    ultrasonography findings, 95f, 96

M
Magnetic resonance imaging
    architectural distortion, in infiltrating ductal carcinoma,
        182f, 188f
    calcifications
        dystrophic, lumpectomy scar and, 40f
        fine linear, in infiltrating ductal carcinoma, 89f
    circumscribed masses, in invasive ductal
        carcinoma, 121f
    irregular masses
        infiltrating ductal carcinoma, 134f, 138f
        inflammatory carcinoma, 144f, 146f
    in mammographic asymmetry
        infiltrating ductal carcinoma, 163f, 165f, 174f
        invasive lobular carcinoma, 172f
        radial sclerosing lesion, 157f
Magnification
    calcifications
        fine linear, in infiltrating ductal carcinoma, 89
        fine pleomorphic, advantages of, 75
        skin, 26, 30
    digital vs. screen-film, 19
    field of view and, 19
    in mass characterization, 90
    in screening exams, 20
    in viewing protocol, 15–16
Magnification compression panel, vs. spot magnification
        paddle, 61
Mammographic asymmetry
    and architectural distortion association, 175
    BI-RADS assessments, 152, 152t
        evaluation methods establishing, 149, 151t
        and follow-up imaging, 152
    causes, 14
    evaluation, 148–149, 150f–151f, 151t–152t, 152
    in fibroadenoma, 154f–155f
    global vs. focal, 148–149
    imaging challenges, 149, 152
    in infiltrating ductal carcinoma, 160f–161f
        after excision of atypical ductal hyperplasia,
            166f–167f
        in elderly woman, 158f–159f
        with outer quadrant thickening, 173f–174f
        with palpable mass, 162f–163f
    in invasive lobular carcinoma, 168f–169f
        diffusely dense, 171f–172f
        in elderly woman, 170f
    in radial sclerosing lesion, 156f–157f
Mammographic densities
    screen-film densities vs., 134
    skin contamination and, 28, 28f

Mammographic masses. *See also* Circumscribed masses;
        Irregular masses
    BI-RADS assessments, 91–92, 91t
    CAD sensitivity, 90
    evaluation, 90–92, 91t
    margin characteristics, 91–92, 91t
    shape categories, 90–91, 91t
    technique, 90
Margin characteristics, of masses, 91–92, 91t
Masses. *See* Circumscribed masses; Irregular masses;
        Mammographic masses
Mastitis
    inflammatory carcinoma vs., 147
    plasma cell, linear calcifications in, 49f
Mediolateral oblique views
    architectural distortion, 176
    asymmetric density and mass localization, 105
    focal asymmetries, 149, 151f, 151t
    screen-film vs. digital, in screening exam, 15
    skin calcifications on, 27
Menopause, fibroadenoma after, 34, 113
Metallic compounds, mammographic density and, 28
Metaplasia, apocrine
    mammography findings, 110f
    ultrasonography findings, 110f, 111
Metaplastic carcinoma
    mammography findings, 122f
    ultrasonography findings, 123f
Microcalcifications
    CAD sensitivity, 90
    digital identification
        hard copy vs. soft copy display, 19
        screen-film vs., 19
    examination, 20
Microcysts
    benign, with fine pleomorphic calcifications, 70f
    milk of calcium within, 29
    punctate calcifications in, 54f
Milk of calcium, defined, 29
Milk of calcium calcifications, 20
    mammography findings, 29, 29f, 30, 30f
MLO views. *See* Mediolateral oblique views
Modulation transfer function, 6, 6f
Mortality, breast cancer, mammography screening
        and, 1
5 Mpixel monitors, 11–12
MTF (modulation transfer function), 6, 6f
Multicentricity, in infiltrating ductal carcinoma, 89

N
Necrosis, high-grade DCIS with, 87, 87f
Nipple-areolar complex, in digital mammography, 14
Nipple inversion
    in inflammatory carcinoma, 143, 144
    with subareolar firmness, 183f
Noise, 6, 6f

O

Oil cysts
  eggshell calcifications in, 41
  fat necrosis and, 42, 43f, 44
  mammography findings, 97f
  ultrasonography findings, 98, 98f

P

Pacemaker, in mammography exam, 99f
PACS (picture archiving and communication system),
  12–13
Palpable mass
  fibroadenoma, 112f, 114f
  infiltrating ductal carcinoma, 131f, 189f–190f
  inflammatory carcinoma, 143f–144f
  invasive papillary carcinoma, 124f, 125
Papillary carcinoma
  central, characteristics of, 125
  intracystic, 126f–127f
  invasive, 124f
Papilloma, with sclerosis, coarse heterogeneous
  calcifications and, 68f
Parenchyma
  masses obscured by, 91, 163
  overlapping, asymmetries and, 165
  surrounding central masses, identification
    of, 163
Parenchymal composition, BI-RADS categories, 2
PASH. See Pseudoangiomatous stromal hyperplasia
Peau d'orange, in inflammatory carcinoma, 143
Phantom, digital vs. screen-film, 19
Picture archiving and communication system,
  12–13
Pixel matrix, digital image, 4, 4f
Pixel monitors, 11–12
Pixels, image size requirements and, 12, 12t
Plasma cell mastitis, linear calcifications in, 49f
Pleomorphic calcifications, fine. See Fine pleomorphic
  calcifications
Popcorn calcifications, in fibroadenoma, 33, 33f
Postprocessing methods, 14–15
Postsurgical lesions
  appearance stabilization, 191
  as irregular masses, 92
Pregnancy, breast cancer in, 182
  postpartum subareolar architectural distortion and,
    181f–182f
Pseudoangiomatous stromal hyperplasia
  mammography findings, 116f, 117
  ultrasonography findings, 116f, 117
Pseudocapsule, in hamartoma appearance, 94
Punctate calcifications, 20–21, 21t
  in atypical ductal hyperplasia, 56f
  in benign fibrocystic tissue, 55, 55f
  in benign fibrosis and microcysts, 54f
  in benign lobules, 48f, 51f, 53f

  DCIS and, 53
  in invasive ductal carcinoma, 57f
    with intraductal component, 58f
  mammography findings, 24f, 27, 27f
  round calcifications vs., 51
  in sclerosing adenosis, 45f
  in skin, 24f, 27, 27f
  suspicious, reasons for, 55

Q

Quantum counting detectors, in digital x-ray system,
  9, 10
Quantum mottle, 7

R

Radial sclerosing lesion (radial scar)
  with architectural distortion, 177, 179f–180f, 194f–195f
  diagnostic challenges, 157
  with mammographic asymmetry, 156f–157f
    vs. architectural distortion, 157
Radiation therapy, recurrent rate for, 65
Radiopacity, of skin products, 28
Range, digital, 5
Rim calcifications, 20
Risk assessment, BI-RADS, 21
Rodlike calcifications. See Linear calcifications, thick
Round calcifications, 20–21, 21t
  ductal neoplasms and, 58
  mammography findings, 24t
    benign lobules and, 46f
    in sclerosing adenosis, 45f
  punctate calcifications vs., 51
  in skin, 24f
  suspicious, reasons for, 55

S

Scanning artifacts, 7
Scar
  with architectural distortion, 178f
  as irregular masses, 92
  from lumpectomy. See Lumpectomy scar
  radial. See Radial sclerosing lesion (radial scar)
Scar marker, in digital examination, 38
Sclerosing adenosis
  fine pleomorphic calcifications and, 71
  mammography findings, 52f
  with punctate calcifications, 45f, 52f
  with round calcifications, 45, 45f
Sclerosis, papilloma with, coarse heterogeneous
  calcifications and, 68f
Screen-film mammography
  breast cancer mortality reduction and, 1
  characteristic curve, digital detector vs., 4–5, 5f
  digital mammography vs.
    densities, 134
    diagnostic sensitivity, 1, 2

Screen-film mammography (*Continued*)
in inflammatory carcinoma, 144
in large breasts, 139
masses, 90
skin calcifications, 14, 24
Screening exams, 14–15
CAD and, 19–20
calcifications in benign lobules and, 48
fine pleomorphic calcifications on, 80f–81f,
81, 84
mass characterization in, magnification and, 90
microcalcifications on, 20
screen-film vs. digital mammography, 1–2
skin calcifications on, 27
Secondary signal noise, 7
Secretory calcifications. *See* Linear calcifications, thick
Selenium, in digital x-ray system, 9
flat-panel detectors, 10
Septation
in metaplastic carcinoma, 123f
simple cyst with, 109f
Signal intensity, 5
Signal-to-noise ratio, 7
Skin, in digital mammography, 14
Skin calcifications, 20
with lucent center, 25f, 26
milk of calcium, 29, 29f, 30, 30f
punctate, 24f, 27, 27f
round, 24f
Skin dimpling, in inframammary fold, 185f
Skin thickening
global asymmetries and, 148
in inflammatory carcinoma, 144
Slot scanning detector, for image acquisition, 9
SNR (signal-to-noise ratio), 7
Solid tumors, recommendations for handling, 127
Sound transmission, invasive malignancies and, 123
Spatial resolution, 6, 6f
Spot compression mammogram
circumscribed mass, 110f
disadvantages, 149
fibroadenoma, 114f
with mammographic asymmetry, 154f
infiltrating ductal carcinoma, 131f, 133f, 137, 137f
in infiltrating ductal carcinoma
with architectural distortion, 187f, 188, 189f
with mammographic asymmetry, 158f, 160f, 161
invasive ductal carcinoma, 121f
invasive papillary carcinoma, 141f
mass margin clarification by, 91
pseudoangiomatous stromal hyperplasia, 116f
radial sclerosing scar, with architectural disortion, 179f
scar, with architectural disortion, 178f
Spot magnification views, 14
dystrophic calcifications, lumpectomy scar and, 37f, 39f
eggshell calcification, 41f

infiltrating ductal carcinoma, 135f, 136
magnification compression vs., 61
Spot mammography, digital vs. screen-film, 19
Stereotaxic biopsy, in infiltrating ductal carcinoma, 139, 139f, 140
fine linear calcifications and, 89
Stitching, 7
Storage, digital images, 7
DICOM and, 11, 12, 12t
PACS and, 12–13
requirements, 12, 12t
Subareolar architectural distortion
identification, 183f, 184
with nipple inversion, 183f
postpartum, 181f–182f
Sunscreen, mammographic density and, 28
Survival rates, in breast cancer with axillary nodal involvement, 138

T
Tattoos, mammographic density and, 28
TDLU (terminal duct lobular unit), atypical ductal hyperplasia and, 56
"Teacup" calcifications, 30f
"Tent sign," 176, 178
Terminal duct lobular unit, atypical ductal hyperplasia and, 56
Tissue density, in BI-RADS assessment, 15f–17f, 17–18, 17t
Trabecular thickening, in inflammatory carcinoma, 144
"Train track" calcifications, 32
Trauma
dystrophic changes from, coarse heterogeneous calcifications and, 67
scarring from, as irregular mass, 92
Triangulation, in subtle architectural distortion, 195

U
Ultrasonography
accuracy in cyst identification, 103
architectural distortion
infiltrating ductal carcinoma, 182f, 185f, 188f, 190f, 193f
invasive ductal carcinoma, 184f
radial sclerosing lesion, 180, 180f, 195f
calcifications
coarse, associated with lumpectomy scar, 40f
fine linear, in infiltrating ductal carcinoma, 89f
circumscribed masses
cysts, 100f, 102, 102f
fibroadenoma, 112f, 114f
lymph node, 95f, 96
oil cysts, 98, 98f
pseudoangiomatous stromal hyperplasia, 116f, 117
irregular masses
ductal carcinoma in situ, 130f

infiltrating ductal carcinoma, 131f, 132, 133f, 135f,
    138f, 140f
inflammatory carcinoma, 143f, 146f
invasive ductal carcinoma, 121f
invasive papillary carcinoma, 124f
mass characterization, 92
mammographic asymmetry
    fibroadenoma, 155f
    infiltrating ductal carcinoma, 159f, 161f, 162f,
        165f–167f, 174f
    invasive lobular carcinoma, 169f, 172f
    radial sclerosing lesion, 156f

V
Vascular calcifications, 20, 31f
    in atherosclerosis, 32f
    characteristics, 31
    in fibroadenoma, 34f
Viewing protocols
    magnification in, 15–16
    in old and current exams, 15

Z
Zinc oxide, mammographic density
        and, 28